Management of Tinnitus
- The Enriching Views of
Treatment Options

Edited by Tang-Chuan Wang

Published in London, United Kingdom

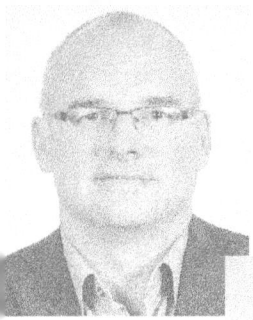
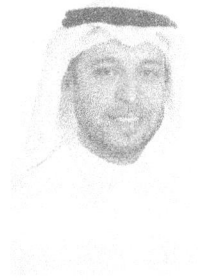
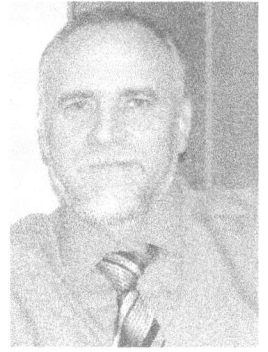
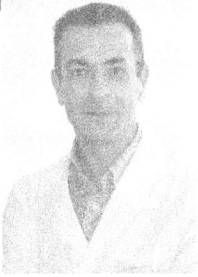
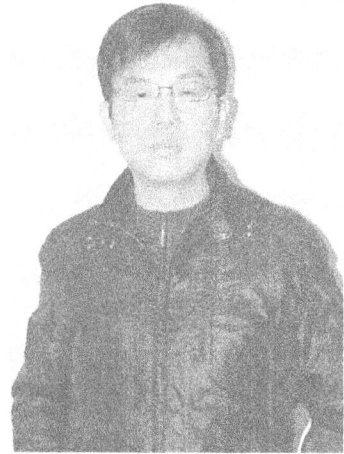
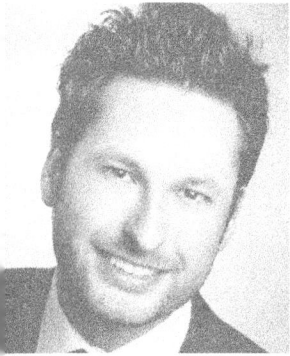
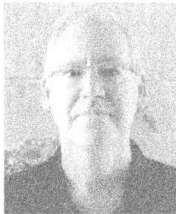

IntechOpen

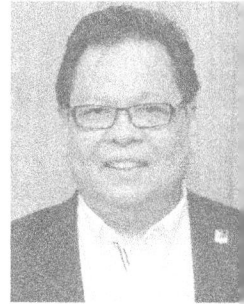
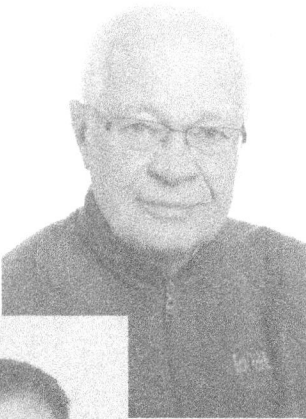
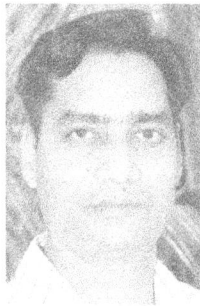
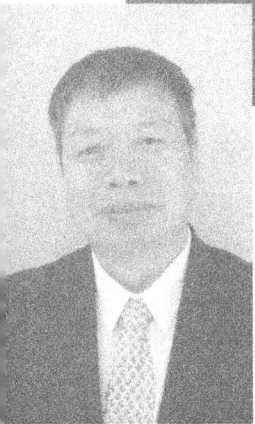
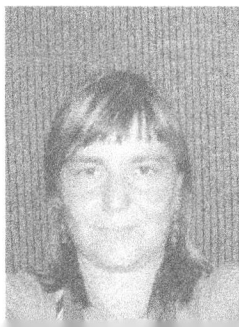
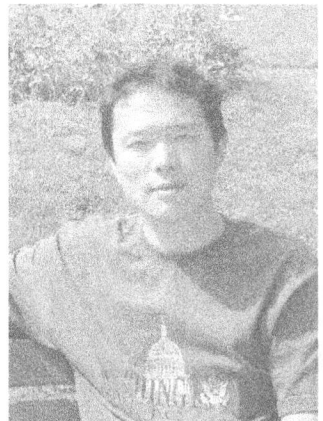

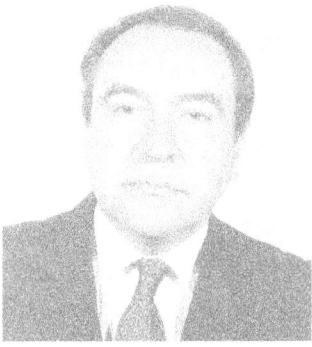

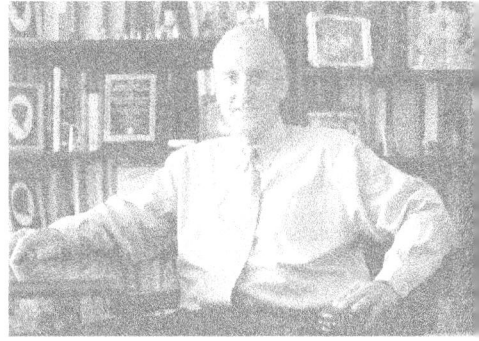

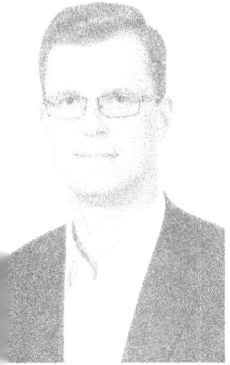

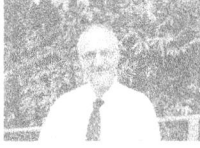

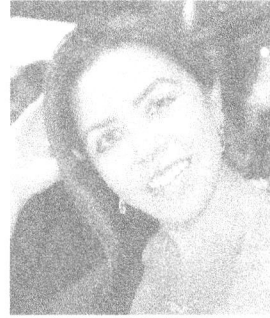

Supporting open minds since 2005

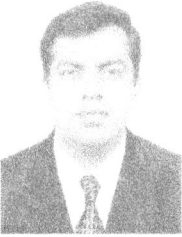

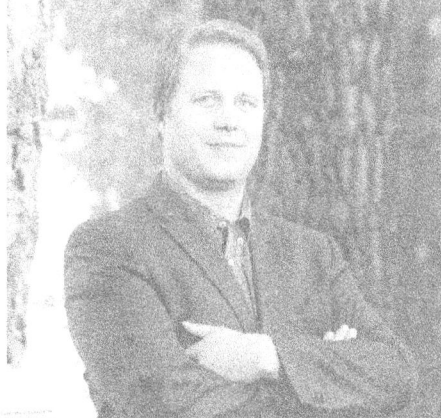

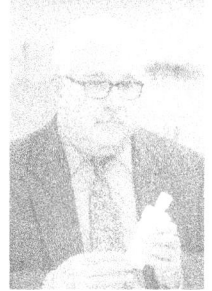

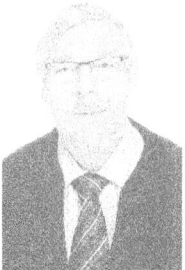

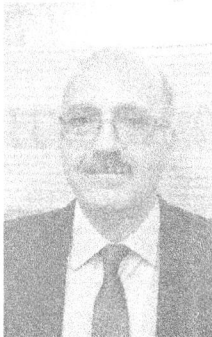

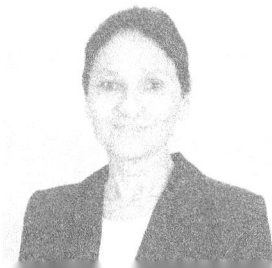

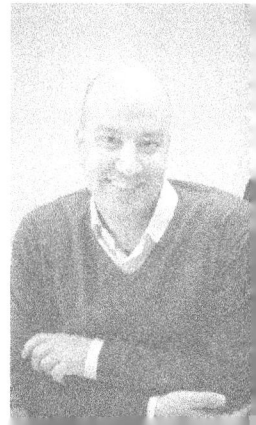

Management of Tinnitus - The Enriching Views of Treatment Options
http://dx.doi.org/10.5772/intechopen.75486
Edited by Tang-Chuan Wang

Contributors
Mohammad Hossein Khosravi, Masoumeh Saeedi, Jaleh Yousefi, Ali Bagherihagh, Elnaz Ahmadzadeh,
İsmail Aytaç, Ayo Osisanya, Henrique Furlan Pauna, Maria Stella Arantes Amaral, Miguel Hyppolito,
Tang-Chuan Wang

Notice
Statements and opinions expressed in the chapters are these of the individual contributors and not
necessarily those of the editors or publisher. No responsibility is accepted for the accuracy of
information contained in the published chapters. The publisher assumes no responsibility for any
damage or injury to persons or property arising out of the use of any materials, instructions, methods
or ideas contained in the book.

First published in London, United Kingdom, 2019 by IntechOpen
IntechOpen is the global imprint of INTECHOPEN LIMITED, registered in England and Wales,
registration number: 11086078, The Shard, 25th floor, 32 London Bridge Street
London, SE19SG - United Kingdom
Printed in Croatia

British Library Cataloguing-in-Publication Data
A catalogue record for this book is available from the British Library

Additional hard and PDF copies can be obtained from orders@intechopen.com

Management of Tinnitus - The Enriching Views of Treatment Options
Edited by Tang-Chuan Wang
p. cm.
Print ISBN 978-1-78985-325-4
Online ISBN 978-1-78985-326-1
eBook (PDF) ISBN 978-1-78985-631-6

We are IntechOpen,
the world's leading publisher of Open Access books
Built by scientists, for scientists

4,200+
Open access books available

116,000+
International authors and editors

125M+
Downloads

Our authors are among the

151
Countries delivered to

Top 1%
most cited scientists

12.2%
Contributors from top 500 universities

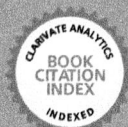

CLARIVATE ANALYTICS
BOOK CITATION INDEX
INDEXED

WEB OF SCIENCE™

Selection of our books indexed in the Book Citation Index
in Web of Science™ Core Collection (BKCI)

Interested in publishing with us?
Contact book.department@intechopen.com

Numbers displayed above are based on latest data collected.
For more information visit www.intechopen.com

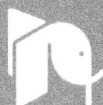

Meet the editor

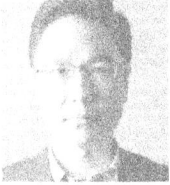

Dr. Tang-Chuan Wang is an excellent otolaryngologist—head and neck surgeon from Taiwan. He is also a research scholar at Harvard Medical School and University of Iowa hospitals. During his Fulbright experience, he worked in Hospital of the University of Pennsylvania, Boston Children's Hospital and Massachusetts Eye and Ear. Besides his great efforts in clinical and basic medicine, he is also branching out into public health in Taiwan. In recent years, he has been devoted to innovation. He always says that "in theoretical or practical aspects, no innovation is a step backward." Due to his contribution to biomedical engineering, he was invited into executive committee of HIWIN-CMU Joint R & D Center in Taiwan.

Contents

Preface

Tinnitus ("ringing in the ears") is a serious health condition that can negatively affect a patient's quality of life. This book provides a multidisciplinary overview on the evaluation and management of this widespread and troubling disorder. Although at present there is no perfect way to cure tinnitus, some good, well-established methods can significantly reduce the burden of tinnitus. Importantly, the only way to success is to take in detailed knowledge of clinicians and researchers. This book incorporates updated developments as well as future perspectives in the ever-expanding field of tinnitus treatment. Because of its organization and its extensive subject index, this book can also serve as a reference for persons who are involved in this field, whether they are clinicians, researchers, or patients. Once we integrate the views of various disciplines and treatment options, we can step forward to manage tinnitus well.

Because there is currently no clinically proven one way to fully eliminate tinnitus for most chronic cases, the ideal treatment option often depends on the various factors of each patient. Therefore, successful management of tinnitus might combine multi-levels of treatment to lessen the burden of tinnitus. In this book, organized sections offer some perspectives from various treatment options, such as sound therapies, temporomandibular joint therapies, herbal therapies, and some alternative therapies. I hope this book helps readers expand the field of tinnitus management.

In the section on sound therapies for elderly patients with hypertension, Dr. Ayo Osisanya discusses the efficacy of audiological tinnitus management options considered essential in the rehabilitation of individuals with comorbidity of hypertension and tinnitus. He highlights the benefits of combined therapies and concludes with some useful recommendations for effective management of the comorbid conditions. In the section on temporomandibular joint (TMJ) therapies, Dr. Henrique F. Pauna et al. presents some TMJ therapies and provides studies that have shown benefits for treating tinnitus associated with temporomandibular disorders. He suggests that TMJ therapies should employ an interdisciplinary approach in order to extend and maximize its effect.

In the section on herbal therapies, Dr. Mohammad Hossein Khosravi et al. talk about current medicinal plants for the treatment of tinnitus; they think that today's world is going toward the use of medicinal plants, and herbal medicine is now finding its place in the market. In the section on complementary and alternative therapies, Dr. Aytaç İsmail will review the complementary and alternative treatments now being used for tinnitus. Through a holistic approach combined with medical know-how, patients can sometimes gain control over their problems, decreasing or even eliminating the effects of these problems. For that reason, the prevalence and acceptance of non-traditional approaches for tinnitus have increased among both patients and practitioners.

I appreciate all those who contributed to this book. Their efforts made possible the success of this academic work. I would like to thank Manuela Gabric and

Kristina Jurdana, the author service managers; Edita Umihanic, the publishing process manager; and Mirena Calmic, the commissioning editor, for their wonderful assistance. In addition, the technical editors were indispensable to the uniform format in this book. At last, I am forever grateful to the persons who raised me well, including my family, teachers, and colleagues.

Tang-Chuan Wang (Vincent Wang)
Chairman of Otolaryngology—Head and Neck Surgery,
China Medical University,
Hsinchu Hospital,
Taiwan

School of Medicine,
China Medical University,
Taiwan

Department of Public Health,
China Medical University,
Taiwan

Research Scholar of Harvard Medical School,
USA

Research Scholar of University of Iowa Hospitals and Clinics,
USA

Fellow of the American College of Surgeons,
USA

Member of American Academy of Otolaryngology—Head and Neck Surgery,
USA

Section 1

Introduction

Chapter 1

Introductory Chapter: Management of Tinnitus - The Views of Various Disciplines

Tang-Chuan Wang and Yi-Chien Ho

1. Why do we need to value tinnitus?

Today, tinnitus has become more common in most modern world. In this case, we assume a huge number of people suffer from tinnitus and they desire to find solutions. Furthermore, suffering from tinnitus can be also related to psychological problem in social life. This means that when tinnitus is ringing for 24 hours a day, then people cannot have a standard quality of life, including sleeping. It also affects communication skills which indicate that tinnitus is usually associated with hearing loss, in a physiological way. However, some clinicians do not realize precisely how important the tinnitus is related with their patients' life and put their life in vicious circle.

2. What is tinnitus?

Tinnitus is a condition where individuals are conscious of a particular sound without outside stimulation. It has been shown that tinnitus is a prevalent issue and common in most societies. More than 40 million people in the United States have experienced tinnitus and are currently suffering from it [1]. Many people experience tinnitus, and it is not only related to aging or auditory pathway but also connected with some negative impacts. It can cause psychological and physical reactions which can reduce their quality of life. Today there are more and more researches suggesting that tinnitus may be connected to aging, auditory pathway, hearing loss, psychological issues, high blood pressure, and cardiovascular diseases. Furthermore, there have been a few cases where tinnitus started after being exposed to extremely loud sounds, which means that the noise exposure also has a high risk of tinnitus.

Besides, in most developed countries, tinnitus is more like a "civilized disease" due to people lifestyles being more and more stressful. Stress will affect psychological health with tinnitus becoming a symptom. This matters not only to elderly groups but also youths. Therefore, it is very important to address tinnitus so that people can understand how important the issue is, in order to reduce the impact of it and enhance the quality of life.

3. Tinnitus treatment in proper

Recently, the treatment can come in many forms, such as sound therapy, counseling, transcranial magnetic stimulation (TMS), transcranial direct current stimulation (tDCS) [2], temporomandibular disorder (TMD) treatment [5], acupuncture, herbal medicine, or other alternative treatments. This is why more and more data have revealed to achieve the aim, getting rid of tinnitus successfully. Typically, counseling and sound therapy can provide a significant reduction to the severity of tinnitus [3]. Those wishing to seek for this kind of treatments are suggested to have an appropriate examination and audiological evaluation before therapy. On the other hand, tinnitus is associated with hearing loss [4]. It is essential to deal with the hearing loss problem while processing the sound therapy.

Moreover, counseling plays a critical role in this process. Counseling will focus on both the psychological and physical impacts; it helps the therapist to comprehend different cases better. The purposes are: Firstly, to classify tinnitus into different groups. Secondly, to design a personal program to reduce the impact of tinnitus. Thirdly, to observe the patients' change, which may include patients' sleeping quality, social life, hearing loss level, diet preference, or exercise habit. Coincidentally, tinnitus can happen in various ways, and it is important to find the main reason first and to mark the effect to make a long-term plan to manage tinnitus. Bothersome tinnitus will cause a severe problem and reduce the quality of life if therapists could not identify it. We also believe that different treatments have their potential to be applied into the different groups of tinnitus patients. In general times, it is not possible to treat all tinnitus patients by only one way.

Author details

Tang-Chuan Wang[1]* and Yi-Chien Ho[2]

1 Department of Otolaryngology-Head and Neck Surgery, China Medical University Hsinchu Hospital, Taiwan

2 Department of Speech Language Pathology and Audiology, National Taipei University of Nursing and Health Sciences, Taiwan

*Address all correspondence to: tangchuan1020@gmail.com

IntechOpen

References

[1] Rauschecker JP, Leaver AM, Muhlau M. Tuning out the noise: Limbic-auditory interactions in tinnitus. Neuron. 2010;**66**(6):819-826

[2] Wang TC et al. Effect of transcranial direct current stimulation in patients with tinnitus: A meta-analysis and systematic review. The Annals of Otology, Rhinology, and Laryngology. 2018;**127**(2):79-88

[3] Jastreboff PJ, Jastreboff MM. Tinnitus retraining therapy (TRT) as a method for treatment of tinnitus and hyperacusis patients. Journal of the American Academy of Audiology. 2000;**11**(3):162-177

[4] Tan CM et al. Tinnitus and patterns of hearing loss. Journal of the Association for Research in Otolaryngology. 2013;**14**(2):275-282

[5] Lee CF, et al. Increased risk of tinnitus in patients with temporomandibular disorder: A retrospective population-based cohort study. European Archives of Oto-Rhino-Laryngology. 2016;**273**(1): 203-208

Section 2

A Perspective of Sound Therapies for Elderly Patients with Hypertension

Audiological Tinnitus Management: An Essential Audiological Protocol for Elderly Patients with Comorbidity of Hypertension and Tinnitus

Ayo Osisanya

Abstract

Elderly population with comorbidity of hypertension and tinnitus is increasing across the world, and the dilemma in the management of such elderly patients across the neurology and audiology/otology clinics seems enormous due to the attendant effects of such health-related comorbid conditions and ageing. This has been observed to have negative effect on the general well-being of quite a number of the elderly patients identified with the comorbid health conditions. It has also increased the tinnitus severity and related psychosocial reactions of the elderly patients. Worse still, the situation causes undulating increase in the prevalence of the comorbid condition of advanced age both male and female irrespective of cultural differences. Due to the aforementioned, this chapter is written with the aim of highlighting the efficacy of audiological tinnitus management options considered essential in the rehabilitation of individuals with comorbidity of hypertension and tinnitus. The chapter also discusses the benefits of combined therapies in rehabilitating elderly patients with comorbidity of hypertension and tinnitus and concluded with some useful recommendations for effective management of the comorbid condition.

Keywords: ageing, audiological rehabilitation, elderly, hypertension, tinnitus

1. Introduction

The synchronous firing of auditory neurons, which always results in tinnitus, has been clinically observed to have a significant relationship with hypertension—the age-related blood pressure (Bp) elevations as a consequence of changes in the arterial structure and physiological functions accompanying ageing. Although the rise in blood pressure (Bp) is not a normal part of ageing, it often occurs as a result of some underlying conditions such as lifestyle factors, diseases and abnormalities that can aggravate (high) blood pressure, leading to severe complications and increased risk of heart disease, stroke and death. Due to multifactorial relationship between hypertension and tinnitus, the incidence of the comorbid conditions in the elderly population is increasing across the globe, even with increased blood pressure level as a consequence of damage to inner ear microcirculation, ototoxic effects of antihypertensive drugs and increased/constant perception of noise generated by the blood vessels. Hypertension is the major risk factor for cardiovascular morbidity and mortality in the elderly population [1]. Hypertension alters cognitive functions of motor and visual acuity as well as auditory performance in the elderly population. It also leads to vascular remoulding by narrowing the lumen and wall thickening. This may affect cerebral blood flow and also disturbs cerebral metabolism and structure. The negative effect of high Bp levels on intellectual performance can also be linked to alterations in the cerebral white matter [2].

Hypertension which is one of the most common clinical conditions affecting older people in this contemporary time accounts for the majority of health-related cases with evidence of increased systolic blood pressure due to advancing age. Thus, a positive association has been observed as regards to the relationship between hypertension and tinnitus. This promotes vascular changes, inner ear microcirculation and tinnitus as noticed. It in turn brings about cochlear microcirculation, resulting in hair cell damage and consequently tinnitus, a common pathophysiological scenario to many conditions such as arterial hypertension, dyslipidaemia, diabetes mellitus, smoking and caffeine abuse [3]. The association between hypertension (especially arterial type) and tinnitus is stronger in older patients and cannot be disassociated from the hearing loss, which is endemic among attendant tinnitus patients [4]. Also, the clinical and psychoacoustic characteristics of tinnitus in hypertensive and normotensive patients seem similar, as well as tinnitus-related distress [4]. The comorbidity and characteristics of the conditions in addition to advancing age can be attributed to the increased complications and attendant effects of the conditions on the elderly patients. This is evident in the galloping increase in the prevalence of elderly patients with comorbidity of hypertension and tinnitus attending neurology and audiology clinics in this contemporary time. Tinnitus has also been reported to be associated with the use of diuretics with low systolic blood pressure. Although the prevalence of tinnitus is observed higher in patients with uncontrolled Bp ($\geq 140 \geq 90$ mmHg) than patients with adequate Bp control (<140/<90 mmHg) [5], the increased prevalence of tinnitus in elderly patients can be as a result of some factors such as hypertension, vascular disease, diabetes and autoimmune and degenerative disorders.

Age-dependent hypertension, with the prolongation of life expectancy, remains one of the major factors causing cardiovascular morbidity, mortality and pulsatile tinnitus. This always affects older people, with the prevalence of 60% among the elderly [5]. Therefore, blood pressure has been observed as an important risk factor in the development of cerebrovascular disease, congestive heart failure and coronary heart disease [6] which is the major cause of continuous ringing in the ear/head of the elderly population. Often, the associated tinnitus, which is not generated by external stimulus, can be classified as auditory and para-auditory tinnitus. The former represents the majority of cases, and the latter is subdivided into muscular tinnitus somatosounds [3]. With the impact of high Bp and the immense amount of blood flowing in and out of the head, tinnitus becomes evident in the humans, causing hearing loss of different degrees and severity, depending on the severity of the blood pressure. This comorbid conditions always make the elderly to experience vascular abnormality, blurred vision, chest pain, reduced anxiety, irritability, reduced cognitive functions, reduced quality of life, depression, poor communication, fatigue, reduced social functions, mood swing, withdrawal syndrome, poor emotional state or health, regular hospital visit and continued use of antidepressants [7]. Therefore, comprehensive management strategy, involving audiological rehabilitation and blood pressure control mechanisms, might be holistically employed, for it will aid the reduction of hearing-loss-induced deficits of function, activity, participation, quality of life through a combination of sensory management, perceptual training, counselling [8], as well as drug management, psychotherapy and physical exercises to regulate the blood pressure and its flow in and out of the brain.

2. Tinnitus: meaning and effects on the elderly population

2.1 Tinnitus: a health-related condition

Tinnitus is an observed condition in which people experience different kinds of auditory sensation without any external stimulation. Tinnitus, as a health-related condition, can be described as an evidence of perception of noise or ringing in the ear/head without external influence or generation (propagation) of sound signal(s). Tinnitus is regarded as the sensation of hearing kind(s) such as ringing, buzzing, hissing, chirping, whistling or other sounds without external sound signal; it is rather a symptom of underlying condition(s) such as age-related hearing loss, drug-related conditions, high blood pressure, ear injury, evidence of accumulated ear wax, cardiovascular disorders or metabolic disorder and/or a circulatory system disorder [7].

Tinnitus is derived from the Latin word *tinnire* which means to ring, and as a condition it is being described as a conscious perception of an auditory sensation in the absence of a corresponding external stimulus. Tinnitus can be subjective, when the experience is of the individual alone, or less commonly, and it can be objective, when an observer can hear the tinnitus. The sensation is generally of an elementary nature as descriptions of hissing, sizzling and ringing are common, although, in some cases, more complex sounds such as voices or music are perceived [9].

Scientifically, tinnitus is regarded as a kind of sensation of sound in the absence of overt acoustic stimulation, and it can be classified according to whether the perceived noise has an identifiable source, for example myoclonic contractions of tensor tympani muscle [10]. Tinnitus is a deafferentation-induced phantom phenomenon characterised by abnormal cerebral synchrony and connectivity, as the reduced or absent afferent cochlear input causes a reorganisation of tonotopic cortical maps, where representations of those frequency regions neighbouring the deafferented part become expanded [11]. Also, tinnitus can be described as a constant ringing, buzzing noise or a high-frequency whistling sound affecting all age groups. Tinnitus may be present all the time, or it may be an occasional phenomenon. This deafferentation-induced phantom phenomenon may vary in pitch from low sound to a very high sequel, with attendant capacity towards interfering in one's ability to concentrate or perceive the actual (intended) sounds or messages.

Tinnitus has been identified as a common symptom associated with ageing health-related conditions. Tinnitus is a continuous ringing in the ear or head without any external corresponding sound signal, which features noise in one ear or both ears or in the middle of the head. At times, it is difficult to pinpoint the site of lesion, but it is a manifestation of malfunction in the processing of auditory signals involving perceptual and psychological components. It is the sensation of any sound perceived in the head or in the ears without an evident of external stimulus. Currently, there is no universal agreeable definition of tinnitus; but some definitions state that it is a phantom auditory sensation [12–14].

Tinnitus ranges from high pitch to low pitch with multiple tones or sounds without tonal quality, but it may be perceived as pulsed, intermittent or continuous noise. This debilitating condition may begin suddenly or gradually, as well as being sensed in one ear (or both ears) or in the head. This health-related condition has been observed to affect 10–33% of the aged population, and it is mostly associated with some psychosocial and health conditions such as anxiety, irritation, annoyance, concentration and insomnia, stroke, rhinosinusitis, diabetes, head injury, hypertension [15] and reduced quality of life [16]. Also, it has been observed that a number of health conditions are capable of causing or worsening tinnitus. The causes include inner ear cell damage, which always affect the random electrical impulses to the brain loading to tinnitus, chronic health conditions/injuries affecting the auditory nerves, exposure to loud noise, age-related hearing loss, head/neck injuries, auditory canal blockage, Meniere's disease, atherosclerosis, malfunction of capillaries (a kind of abnormal connections between arteries and veins) and hypertension as well as other related conditions that can increase blood pressure [7].

Tinnitus noise may be low pitched, mid pitched or high pitched; it may also be one or more components perceived by the patient. Therefore, diagnosis and treatment are majorly based on self-report. It is important to note that tinnitus is neither a disease nor an illness but a symptom to many treatable health conditions. At one time or the other, people may experience ringing in the ears as a result of the usage of certain drugs (antibiotics or aspirin) and/or being exposed to loud noise of 85 dB and above for 8 hours daily and without adequate ear protection and traumatic brain injury, as part of normal ageing process (presbycusis). It can also coexist with some ear problems such as impacted wax, inner ear abnormality, etc. Tinnitus is a prevalent problem and common in all groups, although in the past, it had been considered as a problem of youths, but now it has been discovered that it is more common among the aged [17]. It is estimated that tinnitus affects approximately 50 million people in the United States of America. A similar ratio has been reported in the United Kingdom [18]. In Nigeria, it is mostly associated with treatable health conditions such as otitis media, stroke, rhinosinusitis, diabetes, head injury and hypertension, which affect 10–33% of the population. The association between tinnitus with functional impairment and reduced quality of life highlights the need for its inclusion in any comprehensive medical programme for the elderly, but it cannot be overemphasised [15]. Therefore, people have to be educated on how to take care of their health to prevent any health hazard which can lead to tinnitus and to avoid suffering from ringing in the ear in their old age. People suffering from tinnitus go through tough time as a result of associated psychosocial [emotional and behavioural] problems which include severe headache, negative thoughts, dizziness, hearing problem, anxiety, irritation, annoyance, concentration problem, sleep difficulties, depression and poor attention focus [7]. Studies have shown that the quality of life is reduced in patients suffering from the aforementioned problems [16, 19]. Meanwhile, it is noteworthy that psychoacoustical characterisation of tinnitus cannot fully determine the level of discomfort evoked by this condition. Thus, it has been observed that a person suffering from tinnitus may not be aware of it and may not feel any discomfort occasioned by the affliction, while another person suffering from tinnitus is constantly aware of the difficulty in attention focus, falling asleep, and enjoying life; this is because tinnitus is perceived differently and allows the individual to react to it differently [20].

2.2 Classifications and symptoms of tinnitus

Tinnitus can be classified into four different groups based on its nature and characteristics. Each of these classifications has different characteristics but with similar nature and symptoms. The four classifications would be discussed as follows:

    i. Subjective tinnitus: This is a kind of tinnitus that can only be perceived or heard by the affected person. Scientifically, subjective tinnitus can be defined as an acoustic phantom phenomenon of a perception of sound in the absence of external-physical generated sound signal(s) [7], which is typically initiated by damage to the peripheral hearing system leading to a sequence of structural and functional changes in the central hearing system [21, 22].

Subjective tinnitus is the most common type of tinnitus, and it always occurs as a result of exposure to excessive noise. Most of the times, this type of tinnitus appears and disappears suddenly and may last for a period of time before it disappears. There are two types of subjective tinnitus, which are:

a. Non-pulsatile subjective tinnitus: This can be considered as the most common type of tinnitus and is typically caused by damage to the peripheral hearing system due to undetectable sounds within the central nervous system.

b. Pulsatile subjective tinnitus: This type of subjective tinnitus can also be referred to as vascular or pulse-synchronous tinnitus due to its relationship with disturbances in the blood flow. Pulsatile subjective tinnitus can be explained as a kind of ringing in the ear/head which is perceived as a rhythmic pulsing experience of thumping or whooshing sound due to increased blood flow or narrowing of the opening of the blood vessel.

This rhythmic tinnitus can be caused by several health conditions such as anaemia or an overactive thyroid gland making the blood to flow rapidly and loudly, hardening of the arteries (atherosclerosis), high blood pressure or irregular blood flow in the brain and around the ear leading to pressure or internal noise generation within the central nervous system. Apart from the common signs and symptoms of tinnitus, inflicted individuals with this type of tinnitus will manifest a health condition referred to as idiopathic intracranial hypertension.

ii. Objective tinnitus: This is a kind of tinnitus that can be heard by another person, apart from the sufferers. Objective tinnitus is an uncommon type of tinnitus caused by inner ear structural defects such as hair cell damage, vascular anomalies or repetitive middle ear muscle contractions and presence of chronic recurrent rhinosinusitis leading to Eustachian tube dysfunction. This kind of tinnitus can be easily treated through the treatment of the cause(s) or by avoiding the risk factors.

iii. Neurological tinnitus: Tinnitus can also manifest as a result of neurological disorder(s) which affect the brain auditory functions. This type of tinnitus is rare and can be caused by some neurological diseases such as Meniere's disease.

iv. Somatic tinnitus: This type of tinnitus is classified in line with the manifestation of ringing in the ear/head due to dysfunction along the sensory system. It is purely the ringing in the ear/head as a result of underlying dysfunction of the sensory system.

3. Hypertension: meaning and effects on the elderly

3.1 What is hypertension?

Hypertension is a condition characterised as an abnormality of high blood pressure (HBp), with an evidence of exerted force by the blood against the walls of the blood vessels. Thus, hypertension as a health-related condition is referred to as high blood pressure that can lead to severe-to-profound complications and increased risk of coronary artery diseases, cardiovascular diseases, atherosclerosis and dementia [23]. This high blood pressure (Bp) has been observed affecting 25% of the world's population, and it is the largest single contributor to global mortality [24]. It has also been found to be a significant economic burden to public healthcare providers in most countries of the world, even with improved pharmacological and counselling treatment.

Hypertension is an age-dependent health-related condition, as it is common in people aged 65 and older, and a clinical diagnosis is established by demonstrating a systolic Bp of greater than or equal to 140 mmHg and/or diastolic Bp of greater than or equal to 90 mmHg on at least three different Bp measurements [24, 25]. Hypertension can be confirmed with a repeated blood pressure checkups, based on the manifestation of consistently high blood pressure with a force of the blood flowing against the walls of the blood vessels. At this junction, it is medically defined as a blood pressure higher than 130 over 80 millimetres of mercury (mmHg) [26]. Also, it has been determined by the volume of the blood the heart pumps and the amount of resistance to blood flow in the arteries. For instance, the more blood the heart pumps, the narrower the arteries, and then, the higher the blood pressure will be experienced. Therefore, the long the force of the blood exerted on the arteries, this will automatically lead to high blood pressure, which will eventually cause some health problems if the condition is not controlled early. Once the condition is not adequately controlled, it will lead to serious health challenges including heart attacks, stroke and a state of psychological stress. In determining blood pressure, two (2) numbers have been recorded which are the upper and lower numbers. The upper number is referred to as the systolic pressure that is the pressure exerted during the heartbeat, while the lower number is the diastolic pressure—a kind of pressure evident when the heart is relaxing after the heartbeats. This reading is important and encouraged to be taken repeatedly for appropriate decision and management. Hypertension is the major risk factor for some health-related conditions. Most of the times, it allows cognitive functions, motor and visual sensitivity and auditory performance of the elderly populations who experience the condition.

Hypertension has been observed to always aggravate pre-existent tinnitus through two principal mechanisms: damage to the cochlear microcirculation and to ototoxicity caused by diverse antihypertensive drugs, such as furosemide and beta-blockers, as an electron microscope study revealed that the primary site of cochlear involvements in patients with hypertensive is the stria vascularis, followed by the Corti organ [27]. It has also been observed that there is an increase of extracellular volume generally associated with high sodium retention in hypertension [28, 29]. The prevalence of hypertension and its related condition(s) is increasing. Thus, patients who experience tinnitus often report significant associated morbidities, hypertension, lifestyle detriment, emotional difficulties, sleep deprivation, work hindrance, interference with social interaction, depression, anxiety, insomnia and decreased overall health have been attributed to tinnitus, although causative relations are yet unknown. Patients with tinnitus can have risk of depression, anxiety, and insomnia [30].

3.2 Types, symptoms and causes of hypertension

There are two major types of hypertension. These types will be discussed based on the observable symptoms and causes:

1. Primary hypertension: Primary hypertension is a kind of high blood pressure characterised by a pressure that is not associated with any identifiable

pathological cause. It is the most common type of hypertension, as it accounts for about 95% of the hypertensive cases, and it is more common among the elderly [31]. This primary type of hypertension has non-universally established or agreed known cause(s) but is observed to occur as a result of various factors including obesity, stress, negative lifestyle and other negative psychosocial-related factors and heredity. The observable symptoms include frequent experience and feeling of headaches, tiredness, dizziness and/or nose bleeds and insomnia.

2. Secondary hypertension: This is a kind of high blood pressure that is less common among the aged population. It accounts for about 5% of the hypertensive cases. Secondary hypertension is an abnormality in the arteries supplying blood to the kidney due to an elevation of blood pressure resulting from the underlying cause(s) such as cardiovascular disorder, uncontrolled primary hypertension, loss of elasticity in the arteries, airway obstruction during sleep, hormone abnormalities, tumour of the adrenal glands and drug-related factors [31]. The symptoms of this secondary type of hypertension include very high blood pressure, systolic blood pressure that is over 180 millimetres of mercury (mmHg) or diastolic blood pressure over 120 mmHg, resistant hypertension, central obesity and palpitation.

Other minor types of hypertension are:

a. Isolated systolic hypertension: This is a type of hypertension mostly common in elderly as a result of loss of elasticity in the arteries.

b. Malignant hypertension: This is a type of hypertension common among the younger adults due to prompt and continuous high blood pressure. This comes with evidence of chest pain, regular headache, psychological stress and trauma, blurred vision and numbness in the arms and legs.

c. Resistant hypertension: This is a type of hypertension as a result of a reaction occasioned by the usage of different types of antihypertensive medications. Resistant hypertension is more common in obese and female gender, with an evidence of diabetes and kidney disease.

4. Effects of comorbidity of hypertension and tinnitus on elderly

i. Idiopathic intracranial hypertension promotes the scourge of tinnitus, especially pulse-synchronous tinnitus among the elderly.

ii. The comorbidity of tinnitus and hypertension can promote the complaints of continued whistling, humming or marching noise heard in one ear or both ears that is in synch with a kind of intermittent pulse and clear indication or manifestation of high intracranial pressure compressing the blood vessels. This is always associated with continuous and severe headache and elevated intracranial pressure.

iii. Comorbidity of hypertension and tinnitus brings about the increase in perilymphatic pressure in the elderly due to the increase of extracellular volume associated with high sodium retention in hypertensive health-related condition(s) [3].

iv. Unresolved hypertension and the attendant effect on the general well-being of the elderly can influence negative personality conducts, even with the evidence of increased negative psychological condition or mood swing, sleep deprivation, frustration, anger, feelings of hostility, aggressive depositions, depression, irritation and reduced quality of life.

v. Significant impact on hearing mechanism leading to reduced hearing sensitivity.

vi. Comorbidity of hypertension and tinnitus significantly impairs the quality of life (health, psychosocial, recreational and work-related) of the affected elderly population.

vii. The influence of hypertension induces or aggravates the severity of tinnitus and other related psychosocial and other distressing symptoms and conditions in the elderly.

viii. Hypertension is a major risk factor of tinnitus in the elderly with systemic diseases.

ix. Comorbidity of hypertension and tinnitus promotes continual and spontaneous firing rate of neurons within the central auditory system leading to increased neural synchrony in the firing pattern across neurons in primary auditory cortex and map reorganisation in the auditory modality. This in turn, due to advanced age, brings about increased systolic blood pressure and cochlear microcirculation, resulting in hair cell damage, cardiovascular morbidity, mortality and pulsatile tinnitus and tinnitus-related distress [3, 4]. Consequently, it has been observed that the prevalence of hypertension and tinnitus-related distress is increasing across the globe, as patients who experience tinnitus often report significant associated morbidities, hypertension, lifestyle detriment, emotional difficult, sleep deprivation, depression, anxiety and decreased in overall health, generally associated with high sodium retention in hypertensive condition [28, 30].

5. Signs and symptoms of comorbidity of hypertension and tinnitus

i. Elevation of blood pressure level and regular population of phantom noise (such as ringing, buzzing, hissing, clicking and roaring) in the ear(s)/head. This sound may be constant or intermittent in nature.

ii. Evidence of hearing loss or complaint of reduced auditory sensitivity and high blood pressure.

iii. Regular feeling of dull or severe headache.

iv. Constant pounding in chest, neck and ears.

v. Irregular heartbeat and difficulty in breathing activity.

vi. Regular or continual chest pain.

vii. Vision and visual-related difficulties.

viii. Constant feeling of depression, insomnia, aggressive dispositions and hostility.

ix. Evidence of pulse-synchronous tinnitus and negative personality conducts.

x. Reduced quality of life and feeling of fatigue as well as concentration difficulties.

6. Audiological tinnitus management

6.1 Different audiological tinnitus management (ATM) options for the elderly patients with comorbidity of hypertension and tinnitus

There are several audiological tinnitus management options available towards the rehabilitation of the elderly patients with comorbidity of hypertension and tinnitus. The different ATM options are discussed as follows:

i. Tinnitus retraining therapy (TRT)

Tinnitus retraining therapy is a form of habitual therapy designed to help people who are suffering from tinnitus. TRT is a kind of therapeutic mechanism which is used as a noise generator towards rehabilitating individuals with tinnitus by exposing them to a kind of background noise level towards reducing the negative effect of unwanted sound perception and to also overshadow the perception of the ringing in the ear/head.

Tinnitus retraining therapy is designed to alter the mechanism that transfers the signal from the auditory mechanisms to the limbic and autonomous nervous systems, thereby removing tinnitus-induced reactions [14, 32]. This TRT is a therapeutic mechanism, which always helps an individual with tinnitus to gradually ignore the sound and the associative effects of the tinnitus condition. TRT is used as habitual therapy to give hope to individuals with tinnitus as well as a mechanism of relief to those who are willing to be rehabilitated or adjusted with the condition [33]. Structurally, TRT is designed to help individuals with tinnitus to understand and learn how to stop thinking about the perceived ear/head noise. This therapy makes use of white noise or environmental sounds to block out the tinnitus noise, thereby training the brain to ignore the perception of the negative sound. It is a training or a process of learning how to cope with the perception of the negative sound consciously or subconsciously. As well, TRT is designed to achieve complete habituation of the noise (ringing) perceived in the ear/head practically done through:

a. Monitoring of the patient's daily living habits.

b. The use of a device, normally worn behind the ear, with the capacity to generate broadband noise to divert attention of the patient away from the perception of the negative sound (tinnitus).

c. Introduction of some psychological therapeutic measures for educating the patient to appropriately ignore the tinnitus noise. This is done in addition to some relaxation exercises and giving of stress management counsels, towards eliminating the patient's anxiety and feeling of frustration.

ii. Tinnitus masking therapy (TMT)

Tinnitus masking therapy (TMT) is designed to promote the reduction of audibility of tinnitus by introducing another sound signal through an instrument known as tinnitus masker. The tinnitus masker is used to generate masking noise which can either be applied to the ipsilateral or contralateral ear. The tinnitus masker can also be placed on a bed side for a patient with tinnitus who is experiencing sleeping difficulty [34]. TMT is referred to as sound therapies designed to minimise the contrast between the tinnitus and the surrounding sound, thereby promoting a shift of the patient's focus away from the tinnitus, and to reduce the fatigue and stress occasioned by the tinnitus. TMT involves the use of several devices to produce masking sounds that will interfere with the ringing in the ear. It also means to offer an expected relief to the individuals with severe tinnitus and associated psychosocial reactions.

iii. Cognitive behavioural therapy (CBT)

Cognitive behavioural therapy is another type of audiological rehabilitative mechanism designed to minimise the negative thoughts flowing in the mind of an individual with tinnitus while at the same time changing the person's behaviour towards the tinnitus. CBT is a therapeutic measure to rehabilitate and reduce the effect of tinnitus and its attendant psychosocial reactions by reducing the distress caused by tinnitus. This audiological tinnitus management mechanism makes use of relaxation strategies, cognitive restructuring mechanism of thoughts, reasoning and modified situations to repattern the thoughts and feelings of an individual with tinnitus to acquire essential skills to respond positively to tinnitus and live well-adjusted life, even with the tinnitus condition.

iv. Tinnitus desensitisation therapy (TDT)

Tinnitus desensitisation therapy is a kind of tinnitus therapeutic strategy to desensitise the abnormal processing of negative sound perceived. This is achieved by redirecting the attention (cognitive processing) of the individuals with tinnitus away from the tinnitus-induced signal and enabling the brain to naturally habituate the perceived tinnitus signal.

TDT makes use of directional (specific) counselling signal therapy and relaxation exercises to enable the natural habituation processing of the tinnitus-induced signal.

v. Biofeedback therapy

This is a kind of therapeutic programme structurally designed to rehabilitate individuals with pulse-synchronous tinnitus. Biofeedback therapy is a nondrug-based treatment employed to rehabilitate individual with stress and pain health-related conditions towards alleviating the negative feelings and psychosocial effects of the condition on such individual. Biofeedback therapy is designed to rehabilitate stress-induced health conditions through relaxation methods. The therapy is structured to help individuals with tinnitus to control his/her breathing system, heart rate and involuntary functions so as to reduce the effect of hypertension-related conditions. With this therapy, the elderly with comorbidity of hypertension and tinnitus will be remediated towards the control of all the bodily processes, such as heart rate, breathing system and blood pressure. Also, it will help to aid the rehabilitation reduction of elevated blood pressure, increased body temperature and disruption of brain functions through the promotion of mental and physical-functional activity to even cope with any occasioned stress due to combined effect of hypertension and tinnitus.

vi. Acoustic coordinated reset neuromodulation

The acoustic CR neuromodulation is a well-structured rehabilitative programme based on noninvasive desynchronising stimulation aimed at counteracting a neural synchrony in the individual with pulsatile subjective tinnitus. Acoustic coordinated reset neuromodulation is a kind of rehabilitative mechanism to bring about significant relief of tinnitus symptoms along with a significant decrease of pathological oscillatory activity in a network comprising auditory and nonauditory brain areas which is often accompanied with a significant tinnitus pitch change [34]. The acoustic coordinated reset neuromodulation is used as a therapeutic mechanism towards the reduction in neural synchrony which is considered as a cause of the decrease in the connectivity across the brain areas involved in the larger salience network [35–37]. In essence, this acoustic CR neuromodulation is an essential rehabilitative mechanism for the elderly patients with comorbidity of hypertensive and tinnitus.

vii. Sleep therapy

This is a kind of therapeutic programme which is structured to rehabilitate individuals with sleep disorder. In most cases, tinnitus patients always experience sleep disorder as a result of attendant effect of the health condition on their physical, mental and emotional functioning. The condition may lead to persistent disturbances, depression, anxiety, trauma and sleeplessness.

Sleep disorder often leads to cognitive changes, mental health conditions and daytime distress. As well, tinnitus patient with high blood pressure often experiences poor quality of sleep due to the negative impact of the health condition. This is occasioned by the perception of tinnitus, especially in a quiet environment, and this always affects the sleep patterns and the development of physical discomfort and other related illness. Most of the times, the attendant difficulty often prevents the tinnitus patients from falling asleep. Thus, it is necessary to resolve the sleep difficulty through the development of skills towards the modification of unwanted sleep patterns.

Sleep therapy is a planned psychological treatment to help patients with tinnitus condition to reflect on their beliefs about sleep and negative feeling, as a result of tinnitus and comorbidity of hypertension. Sleep therapy is an effective strategy to resolve sleeping difficulty and attendant anxiety. It is also effective in modifying the emotional responses of patients with tinnitus and comorbidity of hypertension to the health challenges.

viii. Environmental sound enrichment

This is another type of therapeutic programme well structured to rehabilitate individual with tinnitus-related conditions. Environmental sound enrichment is based on the principle of distraction of one sound for the intended sound (message) to be heard or received. This tinnitus management strategy is commonly referred to as sound therapy in the audiology parlance. The sound therapy, which was introduced by Jastreboff and McKinney in 1993, has been an effective mechanism to habituate any disordered auditory system through the use of low-level sounds (sound enrichment) to regulate the auditory functions of any individual with experience of tinnitus. The most effective way for sound therapy is the usage of a kind of sound enrichment suitable (pleasant and well tolerated) to the patient(s) with tinnitus, although some natural background sounds such as recorded traffic noise or music playing functions (instrumental sounds) and sound generators are well encouraged or advised for effective and prompt result.

ix. Relaxation therapeutic exercise

Relaxation therapy is a kind of stress management mechanism to consciously relax the body and mind of any individual with health-related conditions and stress either directly or through guided assistance by initiating calmness into the lives of those who are exposed to it. This therapeutic exercise is aimed at reducing stress symptoms and enables the elderly patients with comorbidity of hypertension and tinnitus enjoy better quality of life and, at the same time, reduce the effect of tinnitus and hypertension.

Relaxation therapy is a designed process to reduce the effects of noise in the ears/head and psychosocial reactions occasioned by the comorbidity of hypertension and tinnitus-related patient cope with everyday stress. For this therapy would help to boost the confidence level of the patients to handle the condition, maintaining normal blood sugar levels and increasing blood flow to the muscles, reducing tension and chronic pain, slowing down the heart rate and breathing rate and lowering the blood pressure, as well as reducing anger and frustration. Relaxation therapy can be achieved through regular deep breathing exercises, relaxing music, mediation and mindfulness exercises.

7. Recommendations

Due to the attendant effects of comorbidity of hypertension and tinnitus on the elderly population, it is noteworthy to make the following recommendations in order to holistically rehabilitate elderly patients with such comorbid health-related condition:

1. Proper screening and diagnosis of the elderly patients with high blood pressure, with the aim of identifying those with comorbid conditions.

2. Hypertensive condition should be properly managed, so as to prevent the development of pulse-synchronous tinnitus and its attendant effect on the general well-being of the elderly population.

3. Behavioural control mechanisms towards the reduction of body mass index and raised blood glucose, alcoholic consumption and poor diet (especially food with high sodium and low in fruit and grains). At the same time, the improvement in physical activity and better lifestyle changes can help to enhance the quality of life.

4. Reduction in the level of exposure to environmental noise and air pollution, as well as other related causative or risk factors of tinnitus and high blood pressure.

5. Combined audiological tinnitus management protocols should be adopted rather than a single therapeutic protocol in managing elderly patients with hypertension-induced tinnitus and other tinnitus severity reactions.

6. Concerted effort should be geared towards prompt and effective treatment as well as the management of tinnitus-induced conditions, high blood pressure, diabetes and noise-induced and ototoxic hearing loss.

7. Noninvasive acoustic coordinated reset (CR) stimulation (neuromodulation) should be employed as a means to replace electrical stimulation bursts, which might be occasioned due to high blood pressure.

8. Proper sound stimulation, counselling and stress reduction strategies should be adopted in supressing tinnitus and its attendant effect on the elderly who presents with comorbidity of hypertension and tinnitus.

9. The usage of combined devices which includes amplification and sound generator capable of producing relaxing fractal tones should be entrenched in the management profile of the elderly patients with comorbid conditions of hypertension and tinnitus.

10. Constant monitoring of the blood pressure level of the elderly population is advocated, and regular audiological assessment is also encouraged.

8. Conclusion

Audiological tinnitus management with the aim of providing appropriate treatment and adjustment for the individual with hearing loss and other conditions occasioned due to the attendant effects of such condition or associated health challenges remains the essential audiological management protocol for the elderly patients with comorbidity of hypertension and tinnitus. Also, it has been established that there is no single therapeutic programme capable of resolving attendant effects occasioned due to comorbidity of hypertension and tinnitus. Therefore, this chapter recommends combined audiological therapies, several psychological measures and regular physical activity in addition to behavioural modification and changes in life styles among the elderly patients with comorbidity of hypertension and tinnitus. Prompt attention must be paid to health conditions relating to unresolved hypertensive condition and its attendant effect on the general well-being of the elderly. Importantly, regular audiological cum and psychological checkups are well encouraged. The mechanism of aural rehabilitation must also be integrated into the audiological tinnitus management for the elderly patients with comorbidity of hypertension and tinnitus. This will promote sensory management towards enhancing auditory functions as well as increase the probability of positive outcomes, which will enable the elderly patients enjoy good quality of life even with the comorbid health-related conditions.

Acknowledgements

The author is grateful to God for the available wisdom and strength. At the same time, I gratefully acknowledge the influence of several audiological rehabilitative and management training programmes cum exposure over the years and the effort of Adenike E. Adesokan towards the arrangement of the manuscript.

Conflict of interest

The author declares no conflict of interest.

Author details

Ayo Osisanya
Audiology and Speech Pathology Unit, Department of Special Education,
University of Ibadan, Ibadan, Nigeria

*Address all correspondence to: ayoosisanya@gmail.com

IntechOpen

References

[1] Vokonas PS, Kannel WB, Cupples LA. Epidemiology and risk of hypertension in the elderly: The Framingham study. Journal of Hypertension. 1988;**6**(supp. 1):S3-S9

[2] Strandgaard S, Paulson OB. Cerebrovascular consequences of hypertension. Lancet. 1994;**344**:519-520

[3] Figueiredo R, LLangguuth B, Mello de Oliveira P, Aparecida de Azevedo A. Tinnitus treatment with memmantine. Otolaryngology and Head and Neck Surgery. 2008;**138**:492-496

[4] Young J, Klag M, Muntner P, Whyte J, Pahor M, Coresh J. Blood pressure and decline in kidney function: Findings from the systolic hypertension in the elderly program (SHEP). Journal of the American Society of Nephrology. 2002;**13**:2776-2782

[5] Borghi C, Brandolini C, Prandin MG, Dormi A, Modugno GC, Pirodda A. Prevalence of tinnitus in patients with hypertension and the impact of different antihypertensive drugs on the incidence of tinnitus: A prospective, single-blind, observational study. Current Therapeutic Research. 2005;**66**(5): 430-432. DOI: 10.1016/j. curtheres.2005.10.001

[6] Ogihara T, Saruta T, Rakugi H. Target blood pressure for treatment of isolated systolic hypertension in the elderly: Valsartan in elderly isolated systolic hypertension study. Hypertension. 2010;**56**:196-202

[7] Osisanya A, Ojetoyinbo A, Olatunde O. Determination of Pulse-synchronous Tinnitus and Personalogical factors among elderly individuals with idiopathic intracranial hypertension in

Nigeria. XI International Tinnitus Seminar Deutsche Tinnitus-Stifung Charite at Berlin, Germany; May 21–24, 2014

[8] Boothroyd A. Adult aural rehabilitation: What is it and does it work? Trends in Amplification. 2001; **11**(2):63-71

[9] Baguley D, McFerran D, Hall D. Tinnitus. Seminar 2013; DOI: 10.106/ S0140-6736[13]60142-7

[10] Landgrebe M et al. Methodological aspects of clinical trials in tinnitus: A proposal for an international standard. Journal of Psychosomatic Research. 2012;**73**(2):112-121

[11] Tass PA, Popovych OP. Unlearning tinnitus-related cerebral synchrony with acoustic coordinated rese stimulation theoretical concept and modelling. Biological Cybernetics. 2012;**106**:27-36. DOI: 10.1007/s00422-012-0479-5

[12] Anderson GH. Effect of age on hypertension; analysis of over 4,800 referred hypertensive patients. Saudi Journal of Kidney Diseases and Transplantation. 1999;**10**:286-297. From http://www.sjkdt.oorg/text.asp?1999/ 10/3/286/37237

[13] Jastreboff PJ. Tinnitus retraining therapy (TRT) as a method for treatment of tinnitus and hyperacusis patients. Journal of the American Academy of Audiology. 2000;**11**:162-177

[14] Lee SY, Kim JH, Hong SH, Lee DS. Roles of cognitive characteristics in tinnitus patient. Journal of Korean Medical Science. 2004;**19**:864-869

[15] Lasisi AO. Tinnitus in the elderly: Profile correlates and impact in the

Nigerian study of ageing. Otolaryngology – Head and Neck Surgery, American Academy of Otolaryngology 2010 and www.news-medical.net

[16] McKerra L. Tinnitus and insomnia. In: Tyler RS, editor. Tinnitus Handbook. United States: Singular, Thompson Learning; 2000. pp. 59-82

[17] Hinchclifee R, Jackson P. Tinnitus in the elderly. In: Hinchcliffe R, editor. Hearing and Balance in the Elderly. Edinburgh: Churchill Livingstone; 1989

[18] Henry JL, Wilson PH. The Psychological Management of Chronic Tinnitus. United States, Boston: Allyn & Bacon Publisher; 2010. pp. 45-49

[19] Bald P, Doree C, Lazzarini R. Anti-depressants for patients with tinnitus. Cochrane Database System. 2006; 253–258(4):CD003853. PMID:17054188

[20] Tyler RS. Tinnitus Treatment Clinical Protocols. New York: Theme Publisher; 2005. pp. 88-90

[21] Saunders JC. The role of central nervous system plasticity in tinnitus. Journal of Communication Disorders. 2007;40:313-334

[22] Eggermont J, Roberts L. The neuroscience of tinnitus. Trends in Neurosciences. 2004;27

[23] Lindsay J, Herbert R, Rockwood K. The Canadian study of health and ageing – Risk factors for vascular dementia. Stroke. 1997;28:526-530

[24] Raymond V, Bakris OGL. Management of hypertension in the elderly population. The Journals of Gerontology: Series A. 2012;67(12): 1343-1351. DOI: 10.1093/gerona/gls148; Published: 22 August 2012

[25] Aronow WS, Fleg JL, Pepine C, et al. ACCF/AHA expert consensus document on hypertension in the elderly: A report of the American College of Cardiology Foundation task force on clinical expert consensus documents. Circulation. 2011; 123:2434-2506

[26] Folmer RL, Griest SE. Tinnitus and insomnia. American Journal of Otolaryngology. 2000;21:287-293

[27] Tachibana M, Yamamichi I, Nakae S. The site of involvement of hypertension within the cochlea. Acta Oto-Laryngologica. 1984;97(3-4): 257-265

[28] Markova M. The cochlea vestibular syndrome in hypertension. Ceskoslovenská Otolaryngologie. 1990; 39(2):80-97

[29] Sarah NA, Algamal AM, Abdelsalam EM. Prevalence of idiopathic tinnitus in patients with hypertension and its impacts on quality of life. Life Science. 2016;13(1):9-15

[30] Fasce E, Flores M, Fasce F. Prevalence of symptoms associated with blood pressure in normal and hypertensive population. Rev Med Chil. 2002;130(2)160-166

[31] Negrila-Mezei A, Enache R, Sarafoleanu C. Tinnitus in elderly population - clinic correlations and impact upon Qol. Journal of Medicine and Life. 2011;4(4)412-416

[32] Jastreboff PJ. Phantom auditory perception (tinnitus) mechanisms of generation and perception. Neuroscience Research. 1995;8:221-254

[33] Henry JA, Jastreboff MM, Jastreboff JP, Schectte MA, Fausti SA. Assessment of patient with tinnitus retraining therapy. Journal of the American Academy of Audiology. 2002;18:143-179

[34] Vernon JA. Treatment of tinnitus. Communicate. 1996;5(4):18-20

[35] Adamachic L, Hauptmann C, Tass PA. Changes of oscillatory activity in pitch processing network and related tinnitus relief induced by acoustic CR neuromodulation. Frontiers in Systems Neuroscience. 2012;**6**:18. Original Research Article 05 April, 2012. DOI: 10.3389/fnsys.2012.00018

[36] Tass P, Adamachic L, Freud H, Von Stackelberg T, Hauptmann C. Counteracting tinnitus by acoustic coordinated reset neuromodulation. Restorative Neurology and Neuroscience. 2012;**30**(2):367-374

[37] Hauptmann C, Tass PA. Restoration of segregated, physiological neuronal connectivity by desynchronizing stimulation. Journal of Neural Engineering. 2010;7:11. 056008

A Perspective of Temporomandibular Joint Therapies

Chapter 3

Temporomandibular Joint Disorders and Tinnitus

Henrique F. Pauna, Maria S.A. Amaral and
Miguel Â. Hyppolito

Abstract

Tinnitus is defined as a sound a person hears that is generated by the body, rather than by outside source. The word tinnitus is derived from the Latin *"tinnire"* meaning "to ring" and is perceived as ringing, buzzing, or hissing in or around the ear(s). Approximately 50 million Americans are affected, while there is a prevalence of 10% in the United Kingdom among adult population. It has multiple etiologies and is sometimes idiopathic. Tinnitus may vary widely to pitch, loudness, description of sound, special localization, and temporal pattern. Most often, tinnitus is associated with other aural symptoms, such as hearing loss and hyperacusis. Tinnitus may result in sleep disturbances, work impairments, distress. Males are more likely to suffer from tinnitus. In the mechanically demanding and biochemically active environment of the temporomandibular joint (TMJ), therapeutic approaches are capable of restoring joint functionality. TMJ treatments including splints, occlusal adjustments, and jaw exercises have been shown to be more effective than no treatment. The following chapter presents a synopsis of etiology, current treatment methods, and the future of tissue engineering for repairing and/or replacing diseased joint components, specifically the mandibular condyle and TMJ disc.

Keywords: tinnitus, temporomandibular joint, anatomical interactions, multidisciplinary approach, hypersensitivity

1. Introduction

Tinnitus is a sensation of sound perceived by the individual regardless of external sound stimulus. It is a symptom present or considered as a manifestation of different diseases. It can be manifested as a simple noise with no clinical complaining, or intense enough to prohibit the social activities of the individual. Up to 50% of cases are tinnitus, the etiology of which is unknown, but often tinnitus is associated with hearing loss, trauma, or ototoxic medication leading to cochlear damage, with sustained neural changes in the central auditory system causing such lesions [1, 2].

The global prevalence of tinnitus reaches 14–32%. It occurs at all ages and increases with aging, which can affect both men and women alike. Approximately 4% of the North American population suffers from a severe form of tinnitus [3, 4]. In a more recent meta-analysis, McCormack et al. found a prevalence of tinnitus ranging from 5.1 to 42.7%. They also found that tinnitus is commonly observed among elderly population (8–20% in individuals above the age of 60 years) [5].

Disabling tinnitus was considered by the "Public Health Agency of America" in 1984 and 1985 to be the third worst condition a person can have [6].

One of the most known classifications to address tinnitus is the one that address to its source of origin. Tinnitus can originate from the sensorineural hearing system and para-auditory system. Tinnitus classified as sensorineural origin occurs due to injury and/or functional breakdown in the sensorineural hearing system, whether in the inner ear or the central auditory pathways. Tinnitus originated from the para-auditory system can be caused by vascular or muscular structures [7].

Tinnitus originated from the sensorineural hearing system is more frequent than the tinnitus originated from the para-auditory system and may be accompanied by a hearing loss (more frequently) or not [8].

2. Physiopathology of tinnitus

The pathophysiology of tinnitus of sensorineural origin has not yet been fully established, although some authors believe that tinnitus would be the result of an exacerbated neuronal activity in the auditory pathways, usually of an excitatory nature, which would be interpreted as sound by the auditory cortex [9].

Both expression and intensity of tinnitus are difficult to quantify, leading to diagnostic, prognostic, and therapeutic difficulties. Several methods of examination, such as clinical and laboratory tests, scales and questionnaires, have been proposed to measure the intensity of tinnitus [10, 11]. However, the internal contradictions of each of these methods, such as the imprecision of the tests, limit the possibility of establishing a safety application tool focused on the manifestation of these symptoms.

In 1995, Zenner and Ernst hypothesized that tinnitus generation was due to cochlear disorders caused by mechanical trauma or altered blood supply, leading to changes in the properties of inner ear hair cells, increasing spontaneous neurotransmission, increasing the activity of the auditory nerve fibers, and, consequently, tinnitus [12]. Henry et al. described that central neuronal activity would be the basis of tinnitus. Deafferentation of the resulting VIII cranial nerve leads to a central increase of upward regulation, thus increasing spontaneous activity, burst activity, and neural synchrony of the central auditory system [13].

Connections between the dorsal column and trigeminal systems, where the projections end in the cochlear nucleus (CN), have been demonstrated [14, 15]. Excitation of the ventral CN (VCN) neurons in the absence of sound upon stimulation of the trigeminal ganglion has also been documented, and others have shown both excitation and inhibition in dorsal CN (DCN) neurons [16, 17].

According to the animal theory proposed by Shore et al., cochlear damage triggers tinnitus by inducing aberrant stimulus to central auditory structures and increasing the spontaneous activity in the DCN and VCN neurons [15, 18]. The study also shows an increased activity in DCN fusiform cells as a result of upregulation of the glutamatergic somatosensory innervation or changes in glycine receptors [19].

Tinnitus can be a manifestation of a turbulent blood flow near to the auditory pathways, caused by a vascular pathology (such as fistulas or aneurysms) [8]. Tinnitus can also be caused by myoclonic activity of the muscles of the middle ear or the palate, or by functional alterations of the stomatognathic system (such as dental problems, alteration of the condyle position, or loss of the dental support). Individuals with temporomandibular disorders (TMDs) may complain of tinnitus in 33–46% of cases [3, 4]. TMD is related to occlusal, emotional, and neuromuscular (in the mastication muscles). TMD pain may be a contributing factor in the generation of tinnitus, with great interest among many areas [4, 20, 21].

The pathophysiology of tinnitus caused by TMD, as well as the pathophysiology of sensorineural tinnitus, is also a controversial subject. Some authors believe that tinnitus caused by TMD could be explained by many craniofacial nociceptive receptors (such as the ones present under the skin, fascia, periosteum, fibrous capsule, and temporomandibular joint (TMJ) ligaments). These receptors would be stimulated by mechanical forces that deform or alter the surrounding tissues resulting from the inflammatory process and ischemia [22, 23]. In addition, it was proposed that innervation plays a role in the vascular tone of cochlear blood vessels and may also provide a pathophysiological explanation for ear manifestations that occur in trigeminal nerve irritation as in TMD and may lead to tinnitus sensation [24, 25, 26].

3. Anatomical relationship of the ear and temporomandibular joint

Temporomandibular joint is a ginglymoarthrodial joint (meaning hinge joint which permits a gliding motion of the surfaces) that allows the movement in one plane—backward and forward. The TMJ forms a bicondylar articulation with an elliptical shape, and its articular surface is covered by a fibrocartilage (**Figure 1**) [27]. Movement is guided by the shape of the bones, muscles, ligaments and also by the occlusion of the teeth.

3.1 Mandibular component

It consists of an ovoid condylar process seated atop a narrow mandibular neck. It is 15–20 mm side to side and 8–10 mm from front to back. Thus, if the long axes of two condyles are extended medially, they meet at approximately the basion on the anterior limit of the foramen magnum, forming an angle that opens toward the front ranging from 145 to 160°. The articular surface lies on its anterosuperior aspect, thus facing the posterior slope of the articular eminence of the temporal bone [27, 28].

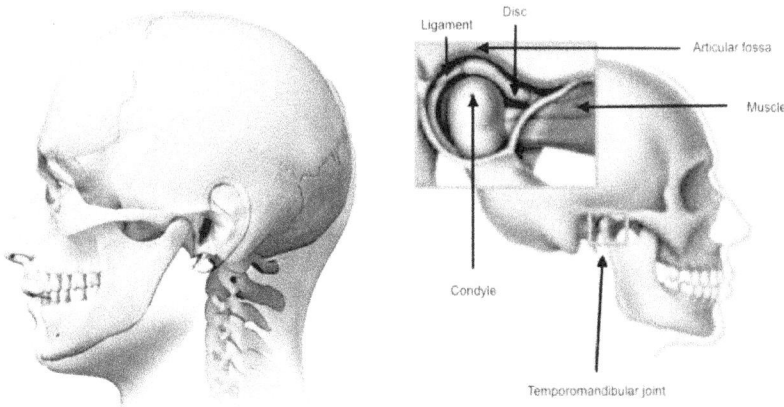

Figure 1.
Left: General picture of the relationship of TMJ and other cranial structures. Right: A closer image of the components of the TMJ.

The mandibular condyle varies greatly among different ages and individuals. Morphologic changes occur based on each individual's development as well as remodeling secondary to malocclusion, trauma, and other developmental abnormalities [28].

3.2 Articular disc

The articular disc is a biconcave fibrocartilaginous structure located between the mandibular condyle and the temporal bone. The articular disc—the most important structure of the TMJ—is an oval fibrous plate. The superior surface of the disc is saddle-shaped to fit into the cranial contour, and the inferior surface is concave to fit against the mandibular condyle.

The disc is attached all around the joint capsule except for the medial and lateral condylar poles, which ensure that it moves in protraction and retraction [29].

Functionally, the condyle and the disc are seated more anteriorly. When the jaw is opened, the condyle moves down and forward (translates). The upper part of the retrodiscal attachment has a rather prominent vascular shunt, and this vascular network is contained within loosely organized fat, collagen, and elastin [30].

3.3 Fibrous capsule

This is a thin tissue completely surrounding the joint. On the lateral part of the joint, the capsule functionally limits the condyle to move forward. This capsule is reinforced more laterally by an external TMJ ligament, which also limits the posterior movement of the condyle.

The synovial membrane covers all the intra-articular surfaces except the pressure-bearing fibrocartilage. The lower and upper compartments form fluid-filled sulci in the joint. These sulci change shape during translatory movements, which requires the synovial membrane to be flexible [31].

3.4 Muscular component

The masticatory muscles surrounding the joint are groups of muscles that contract and relax in harmony so that the jaws function properly. Different muscles are required for the opposite movements of the mandible. These muscles are abductors (jaw openers) and adductors (jaw closers). The temporalis, masseter, and medial pterygoids muscles are adductors, while the lateral pterygoids muscles are the primary abductors of the jaw.

4. Physiopathology of temporomandibular joint disorder

A large percentage of individuals with tinnitus report tinnitus modulation by TMJ and head and neck maneuvers. Up to half the patients who have TMJ dysfunction have tinnitus as one of their symptoms, and in these patients, success rates in eliminating these sounds approach 90%. This suggests that the auditory pathway inputs from the cranial nerves and upper cervical region of the spinal cord are more important in modulating tinnitus than the inputs from the caudal spinal cord [15].

It has been established that, while progressive and regressive, mechanically induced remodeling is a normal process early on. When the capacity for the joint to remodel has been exceeded, remodeling merges into osteoarthritis. Characteristic osteoarthritic changes observed in the TMJ include alterations in shape and overall size of joint components. Degenerative remodeling present in pathologic TMJs may result from either decreased adaptive capacity in the articulating structures or from excessive or sustained physical stress to the articulating structures [32]. Microtrauma of the TMJ (which is caused by bruxism or jaw tightening) or macrotrauma of the TMJ (punch to the jaw or impact in an accident) can lead to muscle inflammation, dislocation of the TMJ, or damage to the cartilaginous disc. Other inflammatory diseases, such as osteoarthritis, may cause degeneration of the cartilage and increased blood flow that may lead to a greater number of inflammatory cells close to the TMJ and the ear. This increase in blood flow may be suggestive of tinnitus perception.

The TMD has as signs and symptoms the limitation of mouth opening, the presence of articular noises during its opening and/or closing, and pain in the musculature of the face and in the TMJ to chew, both uni- and bilaterally. TMD may be presented with chronic pain in the head and neck region, in the cervical region, and the TMJ itself [33].

There are three main theories behind why problems with the TMJ may cause tinnitus or make it worse. Firstly, the chewing muscles are near to some of the muscles that insert into the middle ear (tensor tympani muscle) and so may have an effect on hearing and so may promote tinnitus. Secondly, there can be a direct connection between the ligaments that attach to the jaw and one of the hearing bones that sits in the middle ear. Thirdly, the nerve supply from the TMJ has been shown to have connections with the parts of the brain that are involved with both hearing and the interpretation of sound. The general discomfort associated with TMJ problems can also aggravate any preexisting tinnitus.

Patients with tinnitus and TMD often have excessive somatic concern syndrome with complaints disproportionate to the severity of physical and clinical findings exacerbated by emotional disturbances and are often diagnosed as depression and anxiety. Studies indicate that patients with TMD report their auditory and vestibular symptoms exacerbated, being alleviated by drug treatment and emotional control [34]. These patients demonstrate emotional imbalance, depression, and anxiety. They manifest periods of control of their symptoms. They present physical and cognitive limitations, and the intensity of the symptoms and signs oscillates in an uneven way, suffering the distinct influence of personal, family, professional, and social problems in their daily life [34].

5. TMD diagnosis and complementary tests

The diagnosis of TMD is clinical, being performed through the clinical history and complete physical examination of the joint with palpation, measurement of mouth opening movements, functional tests, and evaluation of joint noises. TMD patients were defined as those who had experience of TMJ symptoms over the previous year as indicated by the presence of one or more of the following symptoms:

a. clicking sounds in the auricular area during the past year,

b. pressure or pain in the auricular area during the past year, or

c. discomfort opening the mouth during the past year [35].

Functional disorders of the masticatory organs are often manifested by acute or chronic pain in and around the TMJ and/or masseter muscles. Impaired dynamics of mandibular movements is manifested as restricted or enhanced range of jaw openings, deviations in the course of abduction and adduction of the mandible, and lack of symmetry of mandibular lateral movements. Acoustic symptoms within the joints, manifested as popping and cracking sounds, are an evidence of the lack of coordination between the articular head TMJ articular discs during mandible movements [2]. Patients with TMD characterize their tinnitus as acute, continuous, sporadic, of short duration, moderate intensity, and that generally did not interfere with their daily activities [36]. Otolaryngological symptoms are a less common group of dysfunction symptoms, including sudden hearing impairment or loss, ear plugging sensation and earache, sore and burning throat, difficulties in swallowing, and vertigo [3, 4, 6].

Due to the latter symptom, patients may experience fear when moving around. Tinnitus may be experienced as squeaks, whistles, chirps, bubbling sounds, pulsations, howls, paper rustle, or sea humming [7]. Facial pain and headache are one of the symptoms of the painful form of the functional dysfunction of the masticatory organ, commonly misdiagnosed and treated as pain of some other etiology [8–10]. The impact of the emotional factors in the development of TMD and common concomitance of otolaryngological symptoms should also be noted. Tinnitus, chronic facial pains, and dysfunctions were commonly reported in depressive patients [10, 12, 13, 37].

Imaging examinations can be performed to confirm the clinical diagnosis, as well as to verify the degree of impairment and integrity of the structures involved. In addition, imaging may also confirm the extent of TMD and assists to document the effects of the treatment already initiated [38, 39].

The imaging tests that may be requested are simple or panoramic X-ray of TMJ, CT, and MRI scans. Both simple radiography and panoramic jaw radiography have low-cost and low-radiation dose but have low sensitivity rates. They are indicated for initial evaluations of less complex symptoms and in the differential diagnosis between TMD and maxillofacial inflammatory conditions [38, 39].

CT scan is considered the "gold standard" for the evaluation of bone structures. This examination is necessary for evaluation in cases of sudden trauma, occlusal changes and limitation of mouth opening, the presence of joint noises, joint systemic diseases, infection, and failure in conservative treatments. Cone-beam computed tomography (CBCT) currently presents an increased indication during the evaluation of TMD [32, 38, 39].

MRI scan has been the method of choice for the study of TMJ pathologic processes involving soft tissues such as discs, ligaments, retrodiscal tissues, intracapsular synovial contents, adjacent masticatory musculature, as well as the cortical and medullary integrity of the bone components, respectively, in the axial, coronal, and sagittal planes, and is highly sensitive for intra-articular degenerative changes [32, 38, 39].

5.1 Electromyography

Electromyography is the study of muscle function, obtained from electrodes placed on the surface of the skin around the muscle, and connected to an equipment for amplification and recording of signals and, therefore, an examination that is capable to verify the action potentials of the muscle fibers of patients. It is considered a safety, easy, and noninvasive method that objectively allows quantification of energy within the studied muscle. It can be useful to assess TMD changes and to follow-up after the established therapy [32, 38, 39].

6. Tinnitus diagnosis and complementary tests

Tinnitus should be evaluated according to a clinical questionnaire, characterizing the type of tinnitus, laterality, continuity, whether there is modulation or not, if there are associated symptoms (hearing loss, vertigo, previous exposure to noisy environments), improvement and worsening, and eating habits, in order to quantify the limitations caused by tinnitus.

The prevalence of TMD was higher in patients with tinnitus and hearing difficulty symptoms than in patients without tinnitus or hearing difficulty, which is consistent with previous TMD studies where reports of auditory complaints are common [35]. Moreover, patients with TMDs were at a greater risk of developing tinnitus and symptoms of a greater severity than patients without TMDs [40]. Excessive mechanical irritation of the disco-mallear ligament is suspected to play a definitive role in the development of tinnitus in TMD patients [41]. Tinnitus has also been linked with pressure and strain from mastication and jaw movement [42]. In an audiological evaluation of aural symptoms in TMD, hearing loss was observed in up to 15–32% of TMD patients [35, 43]. A previous study by Riga et al. attributed the hearing difficulty in TMD cases to increase in resonant frequency in the tympanum ipsilateral to the TMD [44]. The association between tinnitus, hearing difficulty, and TMDs has thus been ascribed to a bidirectional delivery of mechanical stimulation and stress due to anatomical proximity.

TMD prevalence was found to be higher in patients with dizziness/balance disorder than in those without. Otologic complaints most frequently cited with TMDs in the study are dizziness, tinnitus, ear pain, ear fullness, and hearing loss [35]. de Moraes Marchiori et al. reported that patients with TMDs are 2.38 times more likely to present with dizziness, and Chole et al. conducted a case–control study to determine whether dizziness is more common in TMD patients compared to age-matched controls, finding dizziness to be significantly more prevalent in TMD group [3, 45].

The otolaryngological examination should be performed with flexible fibroscopy, verifying the palatal myoclonus. Laboratory tests should be performed with glucose and insulin curves, thyroid function tests, blood count, lipidogram, and audiometric tests (audiometry, impedanciometry, and acuphenometry), electrophysiological examinations (auditory brainstem response, otoacoustic emissions, and eletrocochleography). Cervical spine X-ray, CT of ears, and carotid Doppler can be performed [46].

7. Integrated therapeutic approach

The difficulty of associating tinnitus and TMD is very much associated with the unilateral view of the professionals involved in patient care over the integrated multiprofessional approach [46].

In addition, another difficulty in managing such pathologies is that there is a high number of drugs for the treatment and control of symptoms related to tinnitus and TMD and that have as their side effects the very triggering of these, making diagnosis related to side effects or caused by congenital or acquired disease.

Patients with tinnitus and TMD complaints require careful attention and should be assisted by a multidisciplinary team of dentists, nurses, speech pathologists, ENT doctors, and psychologists. This approach is more effective in diagnosis, therapeutic plan, and prognosis by hierarchizing specific procedures of each professional to approach this patient [15, 46].

8. Results of multidisciplinary approach

Studies have shown benefits for treating tinnitus associated with TMD. Wright and Bifano, in 1997, studied tinnitus in patients with TMD and reported that 56%

were cured and 30% showed significant improvement with cognitive therapy and modulation through maneuvers [47]. Sherman et al. in 2001 found that TMD treatment resulted in greater improvement when combined with psychological and dental treatment, showing improved outcomes when combined with conventional dental therapy alone, implying that psychological factors should be taken into account in the treatment of TMD [48].

Stomatognathic treatment includes therapy of myorelaxant plaques, therapeutic exercises for lower jaw, and occlusal adjustment. Occlusal plaques, considered as reversible and noninvasive devices for the treatment of TMD, can regulate the vertical dimension of occlusion and eliminate malocclusion. They contribute to muscle relaxation, pain relief, and promote neuromuscular stability [49].

Referral to dentists or orthodontists, referral to audiologists, utilization of hearing aids or tinnitus-dampening devices, tinnitus-retaining therapy, music therapy, behavioral therapy related to reducing factors that lead to jaw clenching and bruxism, and osteopathic-manipulative treatment are all therapeutic options that can be considered. In addition, therapeutic options with less of an evidence basis such as acupuncture, tinnitus therapy, hyperbaric oxygen, and others may also be considered for patients who have not responded to other modalities [32, 49, 50].

Treatment through muscle relaxation, through massage and stretching exercises, is reported by some authors. Other authors have shown good results with drug treatment (vasodilators, hemorrhages, calcium-channel blockers, anxiolytics, antiplatelet agents, anticonvulsants, and vitamins) [50]. Okeson et al., comparing muscle relaxation therapies with the use of occlusal plaques, concluded that occlusal plaque therapy was more effective than muscle relaxation therapy in the treatment of temporomandibular disorders [51].

Somatic modulation therapy (treatment aimed at modulating the intensity of a particular symptom, by motion) and electrical stimulation in the treatment of tinnitus have recently been cited. The electrical stimulation of the skin areas near the ear could increase the activation of the dorsal cochlear nucleus through the somatosensory pathway, increasing the inhibitory role of this nucleus in the central nervous system and thus improving tinnitus [52]. For the most debilitating and severe tinnitus, the transcranial stimulation by magnetic stimulation has been studied [53].

9. Prognostic

The increased prevalence of TMD with increased modulation of tinnitus by somatic maneuvers highlights the role of somatosensory afferents, depicting somatosensory tinnitus. However, many questions remain regarding the clinical approach to patients with tinnitus.

1. How close is the association between the capability to modulate tinnitus following somatic maneuvers and the presence of a somatic disorder? The evidence in the study is still scarce.

2. Are there specific individual demographic or tinnitus-related factors that increase the chance of tinnitus modulation? Identification of a tinnitus profile could facilitate patient selection during somatic testing.

3. What is the relationship between tinnitus modulation and the efficacy of somatic treatment? It is hard to hypothesize the relationship of demographic or tinnitus-related factors in patients who are able to modulate their tinnitus,

a characteristic that seems more closely related to somatic components such as the presence of musculoskeletal disorders than to specific demographic profiles.

Current evidence supports a link, mainly for TMD, between the presence of a somatic disorder and higher modulation of tinnitus, especially in patients with a normal hearing threshold.

Identification of specific individual demographic or tinnitus-related factors that increase the chance of tinnitus modulation can be helpful in the management of patients with somatosensory tinnitus. Although some of these treatments may have a positive effect on tinnitus, their effect depends on the correct identification of the underlying somatic disorder, when present.

10. Conclusion

Somatosensory tinnitus is certainly a widespread condition, and further animal studies are required to better understand its pathophysiologic basis. New studies are necessary to investigate whether the correct diagnosis and treatment of a possible underlying somatic disorder could contribute to the management of tinnitus.

Accurate screening for somatosensory modulation of tinnitus is imperative to correctly select patients who would benefit from a multidisciplinary somatic approach. Chronic diseases were associated with a higher TMD prevalence. These findings suggest that TMD treatment should employ an interdisciplinary approach in an effort to extend and maximize its effect.

Conflicts of interest

None to declare.

Author details

Henrique F. Pauna*, Maria S.A. Amaral and Miguel Â. Hyppolito
Department of Ophthalmology, Otolaryngology, Head and Neck Surgery, Ribeirão Preto Medical School, University of São Paulo (FMRP-USP), Ribeirão Preto, São Paulo, Brazil

*Address all correspondence to: h_pauna@hotmail.com

IntechOpen

References

[1] Møller AR. The role of neural plasticity in tinnitus. In: Møller AR, DeRidder D, Langguth B, Kleinjung T, editors. Textbook of Tinnitus. New York: Springer; 2011. pp. 99-102

[2] Langguth B, Kreuzer PM, Kleinjung T, De Ridder D. Tinnitus: Causes and clinical management. Lancet Neurology. 2013;**12**:920-930

[3] Chole RA, Parker WS. Tinnitus and vertigo in patients with temporomandibular disorder. Archives of Otolaryngology – Head & Neck Surgery. 1992;**118**(8):817-821

[4] Pascoal MIN, Rapoport A, Chagas JFS, Pascoal MBN, Costa CC, Magna LA. Prevalência dos sintomas otológicos na desordem temporomandibular: estudo de 126 casos. Brazilian Journal of Otorhinolaryngology. 2001;**67**(5):627-633

[5] McCormack A, Edmondson-Jones M, Somerset S, et al. A systematic review of the reporting of tinnitus prevalence and severity. Hearing Research. 2016;**337**:70-79

[6] Sanchez TG, Bento RF, Miniti A, Câmara J. Zumbido: características e epidemiologia–experiência do Hospital das Clínicas da Faculdade de Medicina da Universidade de São Paulo. Brazilian Journal of Otorhinolaryngology. 1997;**63**(3):229-235

[7] Sanchez TG, Miotto Netto B, Sasaki F, Santoro PP, Bento RF. Zumbidos gerados por alterações vasculares e musculares. International Archives of Otorhinolaryngology. 2000;**4**(4):136-142

[8] Person OC, Féres MCLC, Barcelos CEM, Mendonça RR, Marone MR, Rapoport PB. Zumbido: aspectos etiológicos, fisiopatológicos e descrição de um protocolo de investigação.

Arquivos de Medicina do ABC. 2005;**30**(2):111-118

[9] Jastreboff PJ. Phantom auditory perception (tinnitus): Mechanisms of generation and perception. Neuroscience Research. 1990;**8**:221-254

[10] Sanchez TG, Lorenzi MC, Brandão AL, Bento RF. O zumbido como instrumento de estudo das conexões centrais e da plasticidade do sistema auditivo. Brazilian Journal of Otorhinolaryngology. 2002;**65**(6):839-849

[11] Chen YC, Li X, Liu L, Wang J, Lu CQ, Yang M, Teng GJ. Tinnitus and hyperacusis involve hyperactivity and enhanced connectivity in auditory–limbic–arousal–cerebellarnetwork. eLife. 2015;**4**:e06576

[12] Zenner HP, Ernst A. Cochlear motor tinnitus, transduction tinnitus, and signal transfer tinnitus: Three models of cochlear tinnitus. In: Vernon JA, Moller AR, editors. Mechanisms of Tinnitus. Boston: Allyn and Bacon; 1995. pp. 237-254

[13] Henry JA, Roberts LE, Caspary DM, Theodoroff SM, Salvi RJ. Underlying mechanisms of tinnitus: Review and clinical implications. Journal of the American Academy of Audiology. 2014;**25**(1):5-22

[14] Shore SE, Roberts LE, Langguth B. Maladaptive plasticity in tinnitus–Triggers, mechanisms and treatment. Nature Reviews. Neurology. 2016;**12**:150-160

[15] Ralli M, Greco A, Turchetta R, Altissimi G, Vincentiis M, Cianfrone G. Somatosensory tinnitus: Current evidence and future perspectives. The Journal of International Medical Research. 2017;**45**(3):993-947

[16] Shore SE, El Kashlan H, Lu J. Effects of trigeminal ganglion stimulation on unit activity of ventral cochlear nucleus neurons. Neuroscience. 2003;**119**:1085-1101

[17] Shore SE. Multisensory integration in the dorsal cochlear nucleus: Unit responses to acoustic and trigeminal ganglion stimulation. The European Journal of Neuroscience. 2005;**21**:3334-3348

[18] Shore S, Zhou J, Koehler S. Neural mechanisms underlying somatic tinnitus. Progress in Brain Research. 2007;**166**:107-123

[19] Zeng C, Nannapaneni N, Zhou J, et al. Cochlear damage changes the distribution of vesicular glutamate transporters associated with auditory and nonauditory inputs to the cochlear nucleus. The Journal of Neuroscience. 2009;**29**:4210-4217

[20] Felício CM, Oliveira JAA, Nunes LJ, Jeronymo LFG, Jeronymo RRF. Alterações auditivas relacionadas ao zumbido nos distúrbios otológicose da articulação têmporo-mandibular. Brazilian Journal of Otorhinolaryngology. 1999;**65**(2):141-146

[21] Norena AJ, Farley BJ. Tinnitus-related neural activity: Theories of generation, propagation, and centralization. Hearing Research. 2013;**295**:161-171

[22] Santos Júnior J. Oclusão: aspectos clínicos da dor facial. São Paulo: Meddens;1980

[23] Kaltenbach JA. Tinnitus: Models and mechanisms. Hearing Research. 2011;**276**:52-60

[24] Vass Z, Shore SE, Nuttall AL, Miller JM. Direct evidence of trigeminal innervation of the cochlear blood vessels. Neuroscience. 1998;**84**:559-567

[25] Sobhy OA, Koutb AR, Abdel-Baki FA, Ali TM, El Raffa IZ, Khater AH. Evaluation of aural manifestations in temporomandibular joint dysfunction. Clinical Otolaryngology and Allied Sciences. 2004;**29**(4):382-385

[26] Algieri GMA, Leonardi A, Arangio P, Vellone V, Paolo CD, Cascone P. Tinnitus in temporomandibular joint disorders: Is it a specific somatosensory tinnitus subtype? The International Tinnitus Journal. 2017;**20**(2):83-87

[27] Alomar X, Medrano J, Cabratosa J, Clavero JA, Lorente M, Serra I, Monill JM, Salvador A. Anatomy of the temporomandibular joint. Seminars in Ultrasound, CT and MRI. 2007;**28**:170-183

[28] Yale SH. Radiographic evaluation of the temporomandibular joint. Journal of the American Dental Association (1939). 1969;**79**(1):102-107

[29] Williams PL. Skeletal System. In: Gray's Anatomy. London: Churchill Livingstone; 1999. pp. 578-582

[30] Ferreira LA et al. Diagnóstico das disfunções da articulação temporomandibular: indicação dos exames por imagem. Brazilian Journal of Otorhinolaryngology. 2016;**82**(3):341-352

[31] Toller PA. Temporomandibular capsular rearrangement. The British Journal of Oral Surgery. 1974;**11**(3):207-212

[32] Murphy MK, MacBarb RF, Wong ME, Athanasiou KA. Temporomandibular joint disorders: A review of etiology, clinical management, and tissue engineering strategies. The International Journal of Oral & Maxillofacial Implants. 2013;**28**(6):e393-e414

[33] Pereira KNF, Andrade LLS, Costa MLG, Portal TF. Sinais e

sintomas de pacientes com disfunção temporomandibular. Revista CEFAC. 2005;7(2):221-228

[34] Brown JT, Walker JI. Excessive somatic concern: Diagnostic and treatment issues. In: Walker JI, Brown JT, Galls HA, editors. The Complicated Medical Patient. New York: Human Sciences Press; 1987. pp. 13-30

[35] Song HS, Shin JS, Lee J, Lee YJ, Kim M, Cho JH, Kim KW, Park Y, Song HJ, Park SY, Kim S, Ha IH. Association between temporomandibular disorders, chronic diseases, and ophthalmologic and otolaryngologic disorders in Korean adults: A cross-sectional study. PLoS One. 2018;13(1):e0191336

[36] Morais AA, Gil D. Zumbido em indivíduos sem perda auditiva e sua relação com a disfunção têmporo-mandibular. Brazilian Journal of Otorhinolaryngology. 2012;78(2):59-65

[37] Ferendiuk E, Zajdel K, Pihut M. Incidence of otolaryngological symptoms in patients with temporomandibular joint dysfunctions. BioMed Research International. 2014. ID 824684. DOI: 10.1155/2014/824684

[38] Ormeño G, Miralles R, Santander H, Casassus R, Ferrer P, Pallazi C, Moya H. Body position effects on sternocleidomastoid and masseter EMG pattern activity in patients undergoing occlusal splint therapy. Cranio. 1997;15(4):300-309

[39] Malta J, Campolongo GD, Pessoa de Barros TE, Oliveira RP. Eletromiografia aplicada aos músculos da mastigação. Acta Ortopédica Brasileira. 2006;14(2):106-107

[40] Fernandes G, Siqueira JT, Godoi Goncalves DA, Camparis CM. Association between painful temporomandibular disorders, sleep bruxism and tinnitus. Brazilian Oral Research. 2014;28(1):1-7

[41] Pekkan G, Aksoy S, HekImoglu C, Oghan F. Comparative audiometric evaluation of temporomandibular disorder patients with otological symptoms. Journal of Cranio-Maxillo-Facial Surgery. 2010;38(3):231-234

[42] Pinchoff RJ, Burkard RF, Salvi RJ, Coad ML, Lockwood AH. Modulation of tinnitus by voluntary jaw movements. Otology & Neurotology. 1998;19(6):785-789

[43] Lacout A, Marsot-Dupuch K, Smoker WR, Lasjaunias P. Foramen tympanicum, or foramen of Huschke: Pathologic cases and anatomic CT study. AJNR. American Journal of Neuroradiology. 2005;26(6):1317-1323

[44] Riga M, Xenellis J, Peraki E, Ferekidou E, Korres S. Aural symptoms in patients with temporomandibular joint disorders: Multiple frequency tympanometry provides objective evidence of changes in middle ear impedance. Otology & Neurotology. 2010;31(9):1359-1364

[45] de Moraes Marchiori LL, Oltramari-Navarro PVP, Meneses-Barrivieira CL, Melo JJ, Macedo J, Bruniera JRZ, Gorres VC, Navarro RL. Probable correlation between temporomandibular dysfunction and vertigo in the elderly. International Archives of Otorhinolaryngology. 2014;18(1):49-53

[46] Onishi ET, Coelho CCB, Oiticica J, Figueiredo RR, Guimarães RCC, Sanchez TG, Gürtler AL, Venosa AR, Sampaio ALL, Azevedo AA, Pires APBÁ, Barros BBC, Oliveira CACP, Saba C, Yonamine FK, Medeiros ÍRT, Rosito LPS, Rates MJA, Kii MA, Fávero ML, Santos MAO, Person OC, Ciminelli P, Marcondes RA, Moreira RKP, Torres SMS. Tinnitus and sound intolerance: Evidence and experience of a Brazilian group. Brazilian Journal of Otorhinolaryngology. 2018;84(2):135-149

[47] Wright EF, Bifano SL. Tinnitus improvement through TMD therapy. Journal of the American Dental Association (1939). 1997;**128**:1424-1432

[48] Sherman JJ, Turk DC. Nonpharmacologic approaches to the management of myofascial temporomandibular disorders. Current Pain and Headache Reports. 2001;**5**(5):421-431

[49] Kovaleski WC, De Boever J. Influence of occlusal splints on jaw position and musculature in patients with temporomandibular joint dysfunction. The Journal of Prosthetic Dentistry. 1975;**33**(3):321-327

[50] Herraiz C, Toledano A, Diges I. Trans-electrical nerve stimulation (TENS) for somatic tinnitus. Progress in Brain Research. 2007;**166**:389-394

[51] Okeson JP. Tratamento das desordens da articulação temporomandibular. In: Okeson JP, editor. Tratamento das desordens temporomandibulares e oclusão. 7th ed. Rio de Janeiro: Elsevier; 2013. pp. 317-361

[52] Haider HF, Hoare DJ, Costa RFP, Potgieter I, Kikidis D, Lapira A, Nikitas C, Caria H, Cunha NT, Paço JC. Pathophysiology, diagnosis and treatment of somatosensory tinnitus: A scoping review. Frontiers in Neuroscience. 2017;**28**(11):207

[53] De Ridder D, Vanneste S, Kovacs S, Sunaert S, Menovsky T, van de Heyning P, Moller A. Transcranial magnetic stimulation and extradural electrodes implanted on secondary auditory cortex for tinnitus suppression. Journal of Neurosurgery. 2011;**114**(4):903-911

Section 4

A Perspective of Herbal Therapies

Chapter 4

Herbal Medicine in the Management of Tinnitus

Mohammad Hossein Khosravi, Masoumeh Saeedi,
Jaleh Yousefi, Ali Bagherihagh and Elnaz Ahmadzadeh

Abstract

Tinnitus, which is commonly defined as "ringing in the ears" by the patients, is a perception of an auditory sensation without any accompanying external stimulation. It accounts for a notable part of visits in otolaryngology clinics and has been estimated to involve about 5–15% of adult population making serious problems in 3–5% of patients. Tinnitus causes a lot of problems for patients, their family, and guardians and significantly decreases quality of life of patients. Many treatment methods have been proposed and presented for Tinnitus since the first year of diagnosis. These methods range from conservative management and chemical medications to surgical methods. As the other diseases and conditions, herbal medicine has been trying to treat Tinnitus and a variety of medications have been proposed. In this chapter, we aimed to have a comprehensive review on the current herbal medications of Tinnitus from all over the world.

Keywords: tinnitus, herbal medicine, treatment, epidemiology, *Ginkgo biloba*

1. Tinnitus: definition, etiology, and epidemiology

Tinnitus, which is commonly defined as "ringing in the ears" by the patients, is a perception of an auditory sensation without any accompanying external stimulation [1, 2]. It accounts for a notable part of visit in otolaryngology clinics and has been estimated to involve about 5–15% of adult population making serious problems in 3–5% of patients [1–5].

Tinnitus causes a lot of problems for patients, their family, and guardians and significantly decreases quality of life of patients. Most of the patients have complaints with sleep disorders, depression, decreased self-confidence, and altered social communications as well as difficulties in quotidian activities [2].

Tinnitus is generally categorized into two types: subjective and objective. A majority of patients suffer from a subjective tinnitus, which means perception of an auditory sensation without any evident stimulus. In some patients, a kind of organic measurable stimulus such as glomus tumor, by making turbulence of blood flow, is the cause for tinnitus, which is called objective tinnitus [1, 2]. This type of tinnitus can be found by examiner using an ear-canal microphone or stethoscope [6].

A variety of risk factors have been reported for subjective tinnitus so far; hearing loss, depression, head trauma, and medication-related ototoxicity [7–9]. Some other conditions may have a role in predisposing patients to tinnitus such as acoustic trauma and presbycusis, and it may be associated with temporomandibular joint (TMJ) or cervical spine dysfunctions (somatic tinnitus) as well as depression and anxiety [10–14].

2. Current treatments

Currently, United States Food and Drug Administration (FDA) or the European Medicine Agency has not approved any drug for the treatment of tinnitus [15]. The complex mechanism and innate diversity in etiology of tinnitus have made its treatment a dilemma for physicians and specially otolaryngologists. Despite considerable number of researches, none of the so far presented medications and treatments has resulted in a sustained reduction in perception of tinnitus [16]. No appropriately controlled clinical trials have been successful to prove efficacy of a single drug. Thus, pharmacological treatment of tinnitus seems to be ineffective [17, 18]. Antidepressants are more frequently prescribed for tinnitus and seem to be effective but with a notable number of side effects. Anticonvulsants, benzo-diazepines, lidocaine, and antispasmodics are also among commonly prescribed medications [19]. Voice therapy, using hearing aids, adjuvant therapies as well as environmental sound enrichment are the most common nonmedical approaches to Tinnitus [20].

Regarding the abovementioned issues, there are varieties of complementary and alternative medicine (CAM) treatments, which have been experimented in clinical stage for tinnitus. Herbal medicine or acupuncture, as the most popular types of CAMs therapy among people, have been shown to be effective in management of tinnitus when prescribed solely or in combination [21, 22]. Most of the CAM studies have a small sample size and few methodological pitfalls make it difficult to decide firmly about these treatments.

Some of medicinal herbs and their derivates have been evaluated in various phases of studies: in vitro, in vivo, and even in small to large scale clinical trials [23–30]. In fact, people in different regions of the world have different approaches to medicinal plants and use a variety of herbal medications for treating different diseases and conditions, which have not yet been scientifically assessed [31, 32]. In this chapter, we will discuss and review current traditional and herbal medicine treatments with approved or possible effects on management of Tinnitus.

3. *Ginkgo biloba* (Jinko)

Ginkgo biloba from the Ginkgoaceae family is a Chinese traditional medicine herb, which is being used for the treatment of asthma and bronchitis for a long time [22, 33]. It has gotten popular also in western countries as well as in Asian ones [34]. *Ginkgo biloba* is widely available as easily accessible, inexpensive, and relatively safe leaf extracts with various reported therapeutic benefits such as improved cognition and memory as well as sexual function [35, 36]. These improvements beside other biological effects of Jinko extracts such as improvement of microcirculation and neuroprotection are attributable to flavonoid glycosides and terpene lactones, active pharmacologic gradients of *Ginkgo biloba*. It should be pointed that seeds play a remarkable role in Chinese traditional medicine and they are the most commonly used parts of plants for herbal medications, while *Ginkgo biloba* is processed from the plants' leaves.

Jinko has been proposed for management of various central nervous system pathologies including tinnitus; however, some previous researches have reported no beneficial effects for *Ginkgo biloba* in treatment of tinnitus [36–41]. Nevertheless, no certain decide can be made regarding effects of *Ginkgo biloba* on management of tinnitus according to its complex pharmacological profile, which shows need for further accurate researches [42].

4. Bojungikgitang and banhabaekchulchonmatang (traditional Korean medicine)

Bojungikgitang and banhabaekchulchonmatang have been approved by Korea Food and Drug Administration and are being widely used in Korea for treatment of Tinnitus because of their very low rate of adverse effects [16]. These two herbal medications have found their places among Korean people and physicians. Traditional Korean medicine (TKM) believes that Tinnitus is mainly caused from irregularities in bowel and visceral (zang-fu) functioning [16]. According to TKM, gallbladder deficiency associated with tinnitus is managed by banhabaekchulchonmatang, and bojungikgitang is used to manage the pattern of qi-deficiency [21]. Both of these drugs are now fully covered by Korean National Health Insurance (KNHI).

5. Gushen Pianas

Gushen Pianas is a novel Chinese medicinal herb, which is being used in the treatment of sensorineural hearing loss and Tinnitus. Phlegm-accumulation stasis and splenonephric hypofunction are the two main proposed mechanisms of action for *Gushen Pianas* in treatment of Tinnitus [43]. This medication has been developed by Institute of Otorhinolaryngology of Chinese PLA General Hospital and Wuhan Kexing Biomedical Development Co.

Effectiveness of the drug was evaluated in a phase 2 double-blind randomized clinical trial on 120 patients with sensorineural deafness associated with tinnitus. Patients received five tablets of Gushen Pianas every 8 hours and the effect was assessed after 4 weeks. The findings suggested Gushen Pianas as a suitable treatment for hearing loss with no evident adverse effects [43].

6. *Panax ginseng* (Jinseng)

Root of the *Panax ginseng*, with local name of Jinseng, a Chinese medicinal plant from the Araliaceae family has been being used for treatment of Tinnitus since dawn of traditional medicine [44]. Korean red ginseng (KRG) is a traditional Korean herbal medication, which has been used for more than 2000 years, believed to have several benefits for human body [45]. It is considered that oxidative stress is the cause for idiopathic tinnitus and patients may take benefits from oral antioxidant therapy [46, 47]. So, KRG has been proposed for treatment of tinnitus as it inhibits production of reactive oxygen species (ROS) and also attenuates hydrogen peroxide-induced oxidative stress in human neuroblastoma cells [48, 49]. The effect of KRG (3000 mg/day) was evaluated in a randomized clinical trial in which the patients showed a significant reduction in tinnitus handicap inventory (THI) score and increased quality of life. Also some adverse effects have been reported for Jinseng and specially KRG in literature. Deficiency of vital energy (DE), known as qi-deficiency, is a traditional Chinese medicine syndrome, which indicates the disease emerging identity. Some studies believe that Ginseng, especially Korean Red Ginseng, might cause some adverse effects if the patient's body constitution does not match the qi-deficiency. However, others have reported the Ginseng as the treatment of qi-deficiency caused by any reasons [50].

Further researches are needed to assess beneficial and adverse effects of KRG more accurately.

7. Garlic

Previous conducted researches have reported a lipid-lowering effect for garlic and some others have counted fibrinolytic activity and lowering blood pressure as therapeutic roles of garlic. Few studies have also reported garlic to be beneficial for treatment of tinnitus [6]. Garlic's effect on tinnitus is attributable to improve blood flow of cochlea as a result of its antiplaque formation ability, stabilizing blood pressure, and augmentation in antioxidant capability of the blood. No scientific studies have been conducted for approving these effects and all of them are theoretical [51].

8. Yoku-kan-san

There are more than 120 plants approved by Japanese ministry of health, labor, and welfare, which are now being used in practice as traditional medications [52]. *Yoku-kan-san*, a traditional Japanese herbal medication, is one of these approved herbal medications composed from seven plants (Angelicae Radix, Atractylodis Lanceae Rhizoma, Bupleuri Radix, Poria, Glycyrrhizae Radix, Cnidii Rhizoma, and Uncariae Uncis Cum Ramlus). This combination is more frequently used as treatment of psychological conditions such as irritability, insomnia, night terrors, and hypnic myoclonia, especially in infant patients [53]. Although, there are not enough clinical investigation and convincing data for beneficial effect of *Yoku-kan-san* on tinnitus, but it has been shown to be effective for tinnitus resulted from undifferentiated somatoform disorder in a 44-year-old woman [54]. There is an obvious need for more clinical researches to support such kind of case reports.

Today's world is going toward the use of medicinal plants and herbal medicines, which are now finding their place among people. Conditions with no precise pharmacologic treatment, such as tinnitus, are more probable to be resolved by herbal medications. In this chapter, we tried to review current medicinal plants for treatment of tinnitus; however, currently, there is a lack of clinical research in this issue. The effect of herbal medications on tinnitus should be investigated in more future clinical researches.

Author details

Mohammad Hossein Khosravi[1,2,3*], Masoumeh Saeedi[1,3], Jaleh Yousefi[3],
Ali Bagherihagh[3] and Elnaz Ahmadzadeh[1,4]

1 International Otorhinolaryngology Research Association (IORA), Universal
Scientific Education and Research Network (USERN), Tehran, Iran

2 Student Research Committee, Baqiyatallah University of Medical Sciences,
Tehran, Iran

3 Department of Otorhinolaryngology-Head and Neck Surgery, Faculty of
Medicine, Baqiyatallah University of Medical Sciences, Tehran, Iran

4 Department of Audiology, School of Rehabilitation, Shahid Beheshti University
of Medical Sciences, Tehran, Iran

*Address all correspondence to: dr.mhkhosravi@gmail.com

IntechOpen

References

[1] Michiels S, Naessens S, Van de Heyning P, Braem M, Visscher CM, Gilles A, et al. The effect of physical therapy treatment in patients with subjective tinnitus: A systematic review. Frontiers in Neuroscience. 2016;**10**:545

[2] Baguley D, McFerran D, Hall D. Tinnitus. The Lancet. 2013;**382**(9904):1600-1607

[3] Axelsson A, Ringdahl A. Tinnitus—A study of its prevalence and characteristics. British Journal of Audiology. 1989;**23**(1):53-62

[4] Heller AJ. Classification and epidemiology of tinnitus. Otolaryngologic Clinics of North America. 2003;**36**(2):239-248

[5] Gilles A, De Ridder D, Van Hal G, Wouters K, Punte AK, Van de Heyning P. Prevalence of leisure noise-induced tinnitus and the attitude toward noise in university students. Otology & Neurotology. 2012;**33**(6):899-906

[6] Smith GS, Romanelli-Gobbi M, Gray-Karagrigoriou E, Artz GJ. Complementary and integrative treatments: Tinnitus. Otolaryngologic Clinics of North America. 2013;**46**(3):389-408

[7] Domènech J, Cuchí M, Carulla M. High-frequency hearing loss in patients with tinnitus. Inner Ear Pathobiology. Karger Publishers. 1990;**45**:203-205

[8] Ceranic BJ, Prasher DK, Raglan E, Luxon LM. Tinnitus after head injury: Evidence from otoacoustic emissions. Journal of Neurology, Neurosurgery & Psychiatry. 1998;**65**(4):523-529

[9] Trevis KJ, McLachlan NM, Wilson SJ. Psychological mediators of chronic tinnitus: The critical role of depression. Journal of Affective Disorders. 2016;**204**:234-240

[10] McKenna L, Hallam RS, Hinchcliffef R. The prevalence of psychological disturbance in neuro-otology outpatients. Clinical Otolaryngology. 1991;**16**(5):452-456

[11] Teachey WS, Wijtmans EH, Cardarelli F, Levine RA. Tinnitus of myofascial origin. The International Tinnitus Journal. 2012;**17**(1):70-73

[12] Saldanha ADD, Hilgenberg PB, Pinto LMS, Conti PCR. Are temporomandibular disorders and tinnitus associated? Cranio. 2012;**30**(3):166-171

[13] Abel MD, Levine RA. Muscle contractions and auditory perception in tinnitus patients and nonclinical subjects. Cranio. 2004;**22**(3):181-191

[14] Michiels S, De Hertogh W, Truijen S, Van de Heyning P. Cervical spine dysfunctions in patients with chronic subjective tinnitus. Otology & Neurotology. 2015;**36**(4):741-745

[15] Langguth B, Elgoyhen AB. Emerging Pharmacotherapy of Tinnitus. Taylor & Francis; 2011

[16] Kim N-K, Lee D-H, Lee J-H, Oh Y-L, Yoon I-H, Seo E-S, et al. Bojungikgitang and banhabaekchulchonmatang in adult patients with tinnitus, a randomized, double-blind, three-arm, placebo-controlled trial-study protocol. Trials. 2010;**11**(1):34

[17] Dobie RA. A review of randomized clinical trials in tinnitus. The Laryngoscope. 1999;**109**(8):1202-1211

[18] Lockwood AH. Tinnitus. Neurologic Clinics. 2005;**23**(3):893-900

[19] Mahmoudian-Sani MR, Hashemzadeh-Chaleshtori M, Asadi-Samani M, Luther T. A review of medicinal plants for the treatment

of earache and tinnitus in Iran. The International Tinnitus Journal. 2017;**21**(1):44-49

[20] Ahmad N, Seidman M. Tinnitus in the older adult. Drugs & Aging. 2004;**21**(5):297-305

[21] Kim H-Y, Choi Y-J, Sung E-J, Jo E-H, Kim H-Y, Park M-C. A clinical study of tinnitus. The Journal of Korean Medicine Ophthalmology and Otolaryngology and Dermatology. 2009;**22**(2):139-152

[22] Enrico P, Sirca D, Mereu M. Antioxidants, minerals, vitamins, and herbal remedies in tinnitus therapy. Progress in Brain Research. 2007;**166**:323-330

[23] Samarghandian S, Borji A, Farahmand SK, Afshari R, Davoodi S. *Crocus sativus* L.(saffron) stigma aqueous extract induces apoptosis in alveolar human lung cancer cells through caspase-dependent pathways activation. BioMed Research International. 2013;**2013**

[24] Mansouri E, Asadi-Samani M, Kooti W, Ghasemiboroon M, Ashtary-Larky D, Alamiri F, et al. Anti-fertility effect of hydro-alcoholic extract of fennel (Foeniculum vulgare Mill) seed in male Wistar rats. Journal of Veterinary Research. 2016;**60**(3):357-363

[25] Samini F, Samarghandian S, Borji A, Mohammadi G. Curcumin pretreatment attenuates brain lesion size and improves neurological function following traumatic brain injury in the rat. Pharmacology Biochemistry and Behavior. 2013;**110**:238-244

[26] Moradi M, Karimi A, Alidadi S, Ghasemi-Dehkordi P, Ghaffari-Goosheh M. Cytotoxicity and in vitro antioxidant potential of *Quercus brantii* acorn extract and the corresponding fractions. International Journal of Pharmacognosy and Phytochemical Research. 2016;**8**(4):558-562

[27] Karimi A, Mohammadi-Kamalabadi M, Rafieian-Kopaei M, Amjad L. Determination of antioxidant activity, phenolic contents and antiviral potential of methanol extract of Euphorbia spinidens Bornm (Euphorbiaceae). Tropical Journal of Pharmaceutical Research. 2016;**15**(4):759-764

[28] Karimi A, Moradi M-T, Alidadi S, Hashemi L. Anti-adenovirus activity, antioxidant potential, and phenolic content of black tea (*Camellia sinensis* Kuntze) extract. Journal of Complementary and Integrative Medicine. 2016;**13**(4):357-363

[29] Samarghandian S, Borji A, Hidar Tabasi S. Effects of *Cichorium intybus* linn on blood glucose, lipid constituents and selected oxidative stress parameters in streptozotocin-induced diabetic rats. Cardiovascular & Haematological Disorders-Drug Targets (Formerly Current Drug Targets-Cardiovascular & Hematological Disorders). 2013;**13**(3):231-236

[30] Hajzadeh M, Rajaei Z, Shafiee S, Alavinejhad A, Samarghandian S, Ahmadi M. Effect of barberry fruit (*Berberis vulgaris*) O serum glucose A lipids I streptozotoci-diabetic rats. Pharmacology Online. 2011;**1**:809-817

[31] Samarghandian S, Azimi-Nezhad M, Samini F. Ameliorative effect of saffron aqueous extract on hyperglycemia, hyperlipidemia, and oxidative stress on diabetic encephalopathy in streptozotocin induced experimental diabetes mellitus. BioMed Research International. 2014;**2014**

[32] Bahmani M, Rafieian-Kopaei M, Jeloudari M, Eftekhari Z, Delfan B, Zargaran A, et al. A review of the health effects and uses of drugs of plant licorice (*Glycyrrhiza glabra* L.) in

Iran. Asian Pacific Journal of Tropical Disease. 2014;**4**(S2):S847-S8S9

[33] Khodami N, Shahtoosi M, Amani S, Khodami A. The comparison of *Ginkgo biloba* and Cinnarizine effectiveness in tinnitus intensity of patients with subjective tinnitus. Journal of Birjand University of Medical Sciences. 2015;**21**(4):416-424

[34] Spinella M. The Psychopharmacology of Herbal Medicine: Plant Drugs that Alter Mind, Brain, and Behavior. Cambridge (MA): MIT Press; 2001

[35] Bent S, Goldberg H, Padula A, Avins AL. Spontaneous bleeding associated with *Ginkgo biloba*. Journal of General Internal Medicine. 2005;**20**(7):657-661

[36] Birks J, Grimley Evans J. *Ginkgo biloba* for cognitive impairment and dementia. The Cochrane Library. 2009

[37] Jastreboff PJ, Zhou S, Jastreboff MM, Kwapisz U, Gryczynska U. Attenuation of salicylate-induced tinnitus by *Ginkgo biloba* extract in rats. Audiology and Neurotology. 1997;**2**(4):197-212

[38] Logani S, Chen MC, Tran T, Le T, Raffa RB. Actions of *Ginkgo biloba* related to potential utility for the treatment of conditions involving cerebral hypoxia. Life Sciences. 2000;**67**(12):1389-1396

[39] Maclennan KM, Darlington CL, Smith PF. The CNS effects of *Ginkgo biloba* extracts and ginkgolide B. Progress in Neurobiology. 2002;**67**(3):235-257

[40] Hilton M, Stuart E. *Ginkgo biloba* for tinnitus. Cochrane Database of Systematic Reviews. 2004;**2**

[41] Smith PF, Zheng Y, Darlington CL. *Ginkgo biloba* extracts for

tinnitus: More hype than hope? Journal of Ethnopharmacology. 2005;**100**(1-2):95-99

[42] Drew S, Davies E. Effectiveness of *Ginkgo biloba* in treating tinnitus: Double blind, placebo controlled trial. BMJ. 2001;**322**(7278):73

[43] Zhai S, Fang Y, Yang W, Gu R, Han D, Yang S. Clinical investigation on the beneficial effects of the Chinese medicinal herb Gushen Pian on sensorineural deafness and tinnitus. Cell Biochemistry and Biophysics. 2013;**67**(2):785-793

[44] Salehi Sormaghi MH. Medicinal Plants and Herbal Medicine. Tehran, Iran: The Cultural Institute of Nutrition and Health Press; 2009. chap 1. (In Persian)

[45] Kim TS, Lee HS, Chung JW. The effect of korean red ginseng on symptoms and quality of life in chronic tinnitus: A randomized, open-label pilot study. Journal of Audiology & Otology. 2015;**19**(2):85

[46] Neri S, Mauceri B, Cilio D, Bordonaro F, Messina A, Malaguarnera M, et al. Tinnitus and oxidative stress in a selected series of elderly patients. Archives of Gerontology and Geriatrics. 2002;**35**:219-223

[47] Savastano M, Brescia G, Marioni G. Antioxidant therapy in idiopathic tinnitus: Preliminary outcomes. Archives of Medical Research. 2007;**38**(4):456-459

[48] Cheng Y, SHEN L, ZHANG J. Anti-amnestic and anti-aging effects of ginsenoside Rg1 and Rb1 and its mechanism of action. Acta Pharmacologica Sinica. 2005;**26**(2):143-149

[49] Im GJ, Chang JW, Choi J, Chae SW, Ko EJ, Jung HH. Protective effect of Korean red ginseng extract

on cisplatin ototoxicity in HEI-OC1
auditory cells. Phytotherapy Research.
2010;**24**(4):614-621

[50] Lin H, Pi Z, Men L, Chen W,
Liu Z, Liu Z. Urinary metabonomic
study of *Panax* ginseng in deficiency
of vital energy rat using ultra
performance liquid chromatography
coupled with quadrupole time-of-
flight mass spectrometry. Journal of
Ethnopharmacology. 2016;**184**:10-17

[51] Linde K, ter Riet G, Hondras
M, Vickers A, Saller R, Melchart
D. Systematic reviews of
complementary therapies–An annotated
bibliography. Part 2: Herbal medicine.
BMC Complementary and Alternative
Medicine. 2001;**1**(1):5

[52] Seidman MD, Babu S. Alternative
medications and other treatments
for tinnitus: Facts from fiction.
Otolaryngologic Clinics of North
America. 2003;**36**(2):359-381

[53] Aizawa R, Kanbayashi T, Saito Y,
Ogawa Y, Sugiyama T, Kitajima T, et al.
Effects of Yoku-kan-san-ka-chimpi-
hange on the sleep of normal healthy
adult subjects. Psychiatry and Clinical
Neurosciences. 2002;**56**(3):303-304

[54] Okamoto H, Okami T, Ikeda M,
Takeuchi T. Effects of Yoku-kan-san on
undifferentiated somatoform disorder
with tinnitus. European Psychiatry.
2005;**20**(1):74-75

A Perspective of Complementary and Alternative Therapies

Chapter 5

Complementary and Alternative Treatments for Tinnitus

Ismail Aytaç

Abstract

Tinnitus is described as the perception of sound without any external acoustic stimulation. Any pathology of auditory pathways or any system of the human body may result with tinnitus. The pathophysiology of tinnitus accompanying the disorders of auditory system is not fully understood. In researches, a lot of therapy modalities have been used many years but there is no definitive treatments for tinnitus. Pharmacological treatments of various pharmacological interventions have been investigated for the treatment of tinnitus. However, no drug has been approved by the US Food and Drug Administration (FDA) or the European Medicines Agency (EMA) for the treatment of tinnitus. The use of complementary and alternative medicine (CAM) is very popular in most countries, and several CAM products are often used by individuals with tinnitus with or without medical guidance. Nonconventional approaches for tinnitus have increased in prevalence and acceptance among both patients and practitioners. Many of these approaches have been shown to benefit some tinnitus sufferers. Complementary treatments may be particularly well suited for treating the dysfunction associated with tinnitus, as they specifically target aspects of tinnitus that are often overlooked in conventional medicine. CAM has frequently been used to treat tinnitus. The objective of this review was to assess complementary therapies as a treatment for the tinnitus.

Keywords: tinnitus, treatment, complementary, alternative, therapy

1. Introduction

Tinnitus is a symptom that can be defined as the perception of noise without any external sound source [1]. It is estimated that around 5–15% of the population have a form of tinnitus, and tinnitus may occur at any age. It is more common in elderly individuals (particularly those aged between 60 and 69) than young adults [2]. Many people with tinnitus appear to overcome this situation; nevertheless, tinnitus becomes a serious condition for a 1% minority [3].

However, the physiopathological mechanisms of tinnitus are not well-defined, and this has so far been the biggest challenge in treatment. Broad etiological diversity and symptom subjectivity in the same patient often make it difficult to achieve good results [4]. Moreover, no specific treatment, including drug therapy, is currently accepted as being effective in the treatment of tinnitus symptoms [5].

It is for this reason that patients with tinnitus continue to look for new and more effective treatments. Many of them have turned their attention to complementary and alternative therapies [3].

Complementary and alternative medicine is now frequently being used in the treatment of tinnitus [6].

The increasing popularity of complementary drugs in the treatment of tinnitus requires meticulous assessment and testing of the studies [7].

In this section, we aim to review complementary and alternative treatments that are being used for tinnitus.

2. Methods

Complementary medicine is defined as being a medical practice, or as an intervention, that is sufficiently documented to demonstrate its safety and efficacy in specific diseases and conditions [3]. The standard treatments accepted for tinnitus are as follows: psychotherapeutic interventions such as white noise generators, behavioral/cognitive therapy, hearing aids, benzodiazepines, tricyclic antidepressants, eighth nerve section, and vascular decompression [8].

A range of complementary treatments, such as acupuncture, yoga, homeopathy, hyperbaric oxygen therapy, *Ginkgo biloba*, aromatherapy, and physiotherapy, has been used to reduce the symptoms of tinnitus [9].

2.1 Acupuncture

Complementary and alternative medicine is often used in the treatment of tinnitus, and acupuncture is one of used options [10]. Acupuncture is a method of treatment in which needles are inserted into the body and manipulated. Acupuncture (synonyms: reflexotherapy, sensory stimulation) is defined as the practice of inserting needles into the skin and underlying tissues at precise areas known as points. This is done for therapeutic or preventive purposes. Chinese texts from the first-century BC describe the treatment in systematic detail [11]. The treatment of tinnitus through acupuncture is documented in some books [12, 13]. However, there is still a lack in scientific literature of evidence to support the therapeutic efficacy of acupuncture. Studies have shown that needle stimulation creates an electric charge that has the potential of triggering a rebalancing of the system [14]. Chinese scalp acupuncture is a contemporary acupuncture technique that has been around for just 40 years. It combines traditional Chinese insertion methods with Western medical knowledge of the cerebral cortex. The treatment not only alleviates the signs of tinnitus [15, 16] but also has been proven to be a very effective technique in the treatment of various central nervous system disorders [4].

Studies show that acupuncture enhances tinnitus perception, decreases the intensity of the condition, and improves the quality of life of sufferers. Only a few studies report that acupuncture has a significant effect on the treatment of tinnitus, and these reported effects only provided brief respites of relief [4]. Some study participants demonstrated improvements in sleep quality, blood circulation, and muscle relaxation. After treatment with acupuncture, the subjects demonstrated reductions in the interference of the condition in their quality of life, easy masking by the environment, and forgetting the tinnitus in the presence of normal sounds during daily life more easily [6].

The Chinese scalp acupuncture technique, associated with bilateral electroacupuncture (EA), provided statistically significant improvements in decreasing the intensity level of the tinnitus and also improving a tinnitus patient's quality of life over the short term [6].

A few studies reported that acupuncture could provide immediate relief from both the loudness and discomfort of tinnitus and could thus enable a significant improvement in the patient's quality of life [4]. Other studies failed to demonstrate the efficacy of this approach [17].

Manual acupuncture, electroacupuncture (EA), scalp acupuncture, and ear acupuncture treatments will also be considered as part of the term "acupuncture."

Consequently, in clinical applications, acupuncture treatment applied by experienced and licensed practitioners can be an option for patients with tinnitus. This is especially the case for patients who reject psychosocial behavior therapy, which is the only treatment of which there is clinical evidence of an improvement in the quality of life in tinnitus patients. Additionally, as acupuncture is a safe procedure and there is no current treatment with clinically evidenced efficacy for specific tinnitus symptoms, it is an option for treating tinnitus symptoms in patients who apply to clinics for this procedure [5].

2.2 Yoga

Certain mechanisms of subjective tinnitus are not known, and therefore various treatment modalities are useful in some patients, while they are not used in others. Feelings of depression, a poor quality of life, nervousness, hopelessness, and insomnia in patients are reported, and this situation may change depending on the severity and frequency of the condition. A relationship between tinnitus and the prefrontal cortex and limbic system should be stressed. This part of the brain is linked to emotions. Therefore, when tinnitus is severe, a connection can be made between depression, anxiety, and other psychological disorders [18].

Originating in India, yoga is an ancient and holistic system that includes physical postures (asanas), breathing exercises (pranayama), and meditation (shavasana and yoga nidra). Its name is derived from the Sanskrit word "Yuj," which means to unite, to join, or to add. Yoga is now thought to be the science of existence. The aims of the practice are inner peace and the union of mind, body, and soul. In addition to Ashtanga, Hatha, Karma, Jnana (Gyana), Bhakti, and Kundalini, there are various forms of yoga that enable progress toward these aims. Each discipline is a specific branch of a comprehensive system. Yoga has been reported to decrease sympathetic hormones, stimulate the limbic system, and activate antagonistic neuromuscular systems. Meditation is a hypometabolic state that enables relaxation and reduces the stress caused by sympathetic overactivity. Yoga is reported to play an effective role in reducing stress and anxiety, supporting general health and improving the quality of life [19]. Yoga can reduce stress by certain poses relaxing the muscles of the body and allowing the control of autonomous nervous activity through deep breathing. During meditation, the individual begins a journey toward the inner self. Adopting certain postures allows the body to completely relax, and this helps achieve a higher state of body consciousness.

There are several studies about the therapeutic effects of yoga in cases of conditions such as anxiety, stress, depression, sleep disorders, and stress-related insomnia, as well as hypertension [20].

However, there are few studies in the literature which examine the effect of yoga on tinnitus. Of the studies that do exist, results have shown that yoga exercises performed once a week over 3 months do improve the symptoms of tinnitus. In various studies, yoga has been associated with low levels of stress and anxiety and a high quality of life [21, 22].

Consequently, the findings of studies assert that yoga therapy may play a role in reducing the symptoms of tinnitus [23].

2.3 Biofeedback-neurofeedback

2.3.1 Biofeedback

Biofeedback is a process of learning that influences the individual's physiological processes and aims to provide the best improvements in health [24, 25]. Biofeedback provides information regarding the current state of an individual's physiological process. This allows the individual to learn to appreciate their individual status. The purpose of biofeedback is to allow the individual more control or influence over the progression of that system [24, 25]. One of the unique characteristics of biofeedback is that the process establishes a connection between the individual's mind and body [24, 26]. Individuals are usually unaware of the status of their physiological systems.

However, through biofeedback, individuals are given the opportunity of learning how cognitive and emotional processes affect their physiological functions. When individuals realize that they are nervous, they then can influence this physiological system. For instance, during biofeedback, the instance of muscle strain might be used to help individuals recognize that they are nervous or stressed. Thanks to biofeedback, the individual who requests feedback has the opportunity of seeing the effect of relaxation techniques on muscle strains.

Being able to affect the progress of a physiological system is called "self-regulation" [25, 26]. Learning how to affect one's own physiological functions encourages the individuals to play a more active role in their own healthcare and maintaining a healthy life [24, 26].

Biofeedback is used in the treatment of medical and mental disorders such as anxiety, hypertension, and headache. Additionally, biofeedback is sometimes used as an adjuvant to drug therapy and alcohol treatment. Furthermore, biofeedback techniques are used to not only improve sports performance but also increase optimal functionality [24, 26]. Studies conducted by Sherma (2004) support the activity of biofeedback in many medical and mental disorders [25].

2.3.2 Neurofeedback

Tinnitus is a subjective auditory perception without any physical external source. While it is known that there is a correlation between tinnitus and cochlear damage, its neurophysiology is not currently known, despite the demonstration of some correlations [27]. Damaged hair cells in the cochlea may cause an absence of neurons in the auditory system and the rearrangement of cortical maps [28, 29]. Cortical neurons, which lack certain frequencies, might become more sensitive to close frequencies [30]. Because of this hypothesis, Dohrmann et al. used auto-activity models of the brain's non-auditory and noncellular regions for testing. They did this by using magnetoencephalography (MEG) and electroencephalography (EEG) in patients with chronic tinnitus [31]. They found that the reduced power within the delta interval (1.5–4 Hz) and the alpha frequency band (8–12 Hz) was most distinct in the brain's temporal region. They therefore referred to 8–12 Hz activity as tau activity [32].

Modification of the electrophysiological properties of brain activity may actually affect tinnitus. Neurofeedback has been shown to lead to such electrophysiological modifications [33]. Biofeedback-relaxation training has been assessed for chronic tinnitus [34], and a recent study reports significant improvements in tinnitus distress following a biofeedback-based behavioral treatment [35]. These results might be attributable to biofeedback treatment as electromyography (EMG) parameters remain stable for a period of 3 months [36]. Also, some authors used the relationship between stress, the reduced alpha band, and increased beta band in terms of neurofeedback [37, 38]. It was seen that neurofeedback again increased alpha rhythm and decreased beta rhythm in tinnitus patients.

Similar results were found also in a recent study [39]. A distinct decrease in alpha band (8–12 Hz) and a significant increase in gamma frequency (48–54 Hz), compared to controls, were seen in tinnitus patients [40].

According to a study, tinnitus-related problems in patients decreased following training and in the following months, despite a negligible increase in the tau/delta ratio. It can be concluded that the effects of neurofeedback treatment on tinnitus are enabled by other factors such as placebo, distraction from tinnitus through neurofeedback, etc. However, contrary to the placebo hypothesis in this study, significant results were achieved with patients who received up to 6 months post-treatment, indicating that the results should decrease over time. Stable long-term results for both tinnitus disorder and tinnitus-related problems were also reported in a randomized controlled study of biofeedback-based behavioral treatment [35]. The authors reported improvements in self-efficacy and coping abilities. The effects of neurofeedback on tinnitus comorbidities are therefore seen to be important.

As suggested by Weise et al., a decrease in tinnitus discomfort may be associated with control and emotional control created by neurofeedback [35]. The positive effect of neurofeedback may also be related to the rearrangement of cortical maps [41].

2.4 Hypnotherapy

Hypnotherapy is an altered state of consciousness that allows the subconscious mind to be more open to selective and positive suggestion. It can be very effective in coping with the psychological aspects of tinnitus such as anger, stress, and anxiety.

Hypnotherapy is able to involve various techniques by helping patients feel more comfortable with noise. In order to process tinnitus sounds, the subconscious is able to use sounds produced through hypnosis to make tinnitus less threatening and easier to live with by directing the mind in the same way as background noise does.

By working with the mind (particularly with the part of the subconscious that stores memory, imagination, and behaviors), hypnotherapy may help train the brain and change patients' reactions to tinnitus. An improvement can be achieved in other healthcare problems related to tinnitus by changing the way the mind reacts to tinnitus sounds [42].

This therapy aims to create a deep state of relaxation while protecting normal mental activity. It also allows for better implementation of cognitive-behavioral therapy and some psychological techniques. Modern practice focuses on the studies of Milton Erickson [43], who, derived from many practical techniques, was a keen advocate of the superiority of indirect over direct suggestion. Its efficacy has been evidenced in a series of clinical cases for various conditions, ranging from irritable bowel syndrome [44] to preoperative anxiety [45]. Meta-analysis demonstrates enhanced results for cognitive-behavioral therapy when it is used as a supporting treatment [46].

Auditory cores of the midbrain receive a significant amount of afferents from high centers [47], and subjective experiences of sensory phenomena are modulated to produce striking effects that may cause changes in the levels of auditory cortex activity [48]. Also, as in all chronic disorders, personal perceptions of tinnitus by the affected patient have a strong influence on his/her life. In the light of these two ideas, it can be expected that tinnitus would be suitable for a psychological approach, and indeed, most hypnotherapists consider tinnitus as a treatable condition.

Using hypnosis in the management of tinnitus is not a new concept. Some techniques and case reports which have been debated for over 30 years were published in the literature 20 years ago. Despite hypnosis having quite a long history, few peer-reviewed studies have been conducted on the suitability of various techniques and even the validity of hypnosis as a management strategy. In cases where such a study is present, it is difficult to make a comparative evaluation as there is no standard agreed treatment method. While some individuals assert that tinnitus might be related to chronic pain and treated this way, others use time regression to take the patient back to a time before the onset of tinnitus. Other approaches are to emphasize a session-based approach or the use of self-hypnosis [49].

Hypnotic inner absorption involves concentration and focused attention. When the mind is engaged and focused in this way, it can lead to changes through the use of mind power. The use of hypnosis and self-hypnosis may allow people to gain more control over their behaviors, thoughts, emotional reactions, and even their physiological reactions and physical health.

One study shows that although tinnitus was not altered in 5 of 14 patients, hypnosis did lead to lead to slight relief and reports of the noise being more bearable in the others. There was no improvement in tinnitus matching levels or visual analogue scales in one patient. In another study by Mason, there was no difference between two groups in terms of tinnitus loudness, tinnitus severity, linear analogue scale, and the need for further treatment. The main benefit of hypnotherapy is the fact that it can provide relief and sense of relaxation, making tinnitus more bearable [3].

2.5 Hyperbaric oxygen treatment

Tinnitus is the perception of sound in the absence of evident acoustic stimulation. There are traditional medical treatments for tinnitus; however, they have not proven to be satisfactory. As an alternative therapy, hyperbaric oxygen (HBO2) treatment may improve tinnitus, but benefits provided are not clear [50].

Hyperbaric oxygenation permits a controlled increase in the partial oxygen pressure of the blood. This technique can be used for tinnitus and sudden deafness, which has been caused by the development of a lack of oxygen in the inner ear and brain, and the resulting limited energy supply. Current results support the implementation of hyperbaric oxygen treatment as an alternative therapy when standard treatments fail. Some studies have reported an improvement of 60–65% in tinnitus with hyperbaric oxygen treatment. HBO treatment should be initiated at the earliest opportunity, particularly in tinnitus cases that are accompanied by a sudden loss in hearing. Treatment success in case of sudden deafness depends on the rapid application of HBO. HBO treatment extends the range of treatment possibilities for tinnitus and sudden deafness [51].

2.6 Homeopathy

Tinnitus is a common condition that lacks a practical and effective pharmacological treatment. When tinnitus cannot be overcome through traditional means, patients increasingly turn toward "alternative" or "complementary" drugs [52].

Through the use of a "satisfying dose" for treatment purposes, homeopathic principles may use large "homeopathic" doses of a substance that triggers a symptom in order to stimulate a physiological reaction against the symptoms, thereby eliminating the discomfort. Substances in "active" homeopathic (D60) tablets include pharmacological doses of tinnitogenic medicines such as sodium salicylate, ascaridole, conine, and quinine [3].

In a study, despite survey results showing the preference of homeopathic preparations over placebo in 14 of 28 subjects, a variance analysis showed that neither VAS scores nor audiological measurements could provide significant improvements in tinnitus symptoms as a response to tinnitus. It could not be shown that homeopathy was more effective than the equivalent placebo in the treatment of tinnitus [52].

In another work, results of a placebo-controlled randomized study were published. A study by Simpson on tinnitus disorder, awareness, loudness, and audiological measurements (narrow-band masking) did not show any difference between the groups treated with homeopathic preparations, including sodium salicylate, ascaridole, conine, and quinine and placebo [3].

2.7 Low-power laser

A low-power laser (LPL), with the power of around 1% of a surgical laser, has been reported to be able to accelerate the healing of injured peripheral nerves and soft tissues and to reduce inflammation and pain [53]. Many studies have revealed that the primary absorption area of LPL within a neuron was probably mitochondrion. When laser light is absorbed, protons are released from the mitochondrion to the cytoplasm. It is thought that protons suppress the permeability of sodium and potassium channels that decrease the frequency of nerve action potential. In animal experiments, the compound action potential of the eighth nerve was suppressed by the irradiation of LPL, through a round window directly to the cochlea [53]. The wavelengths used are between 810 and 890 nm within the interval of 40–60 mW. They are passed through the external auditory canal toward the cochlea.

Three studies have failed to demonstrate a significant response to low-power laser [54].

In a study conducted in 2002, active or placebo laser treatment was transmissionally applied for 6 minutes once a week to 68 ears in 45 patients with unilateral or bilateral tinnitus. Laser was applied four times for a period of 4 weeks. A survey was conducted to evaluate the loudness, duration, quality, and discomfort of tinnitus before and after irradiation. Loudness and pitch match were obtained for tinnitus, and auto-acoustic emissions were also examined. No significant difference was observed between active and placebo laser groups in terms of loudness, duration, quality, and the level of discomfort of tinnitus. One patient had acute hearing loss after the third irradiation of active laser treatment. In consequence, transmeatal low-power laser irradiation with 60 mW is not as effective in tinnitus treatment [54].

Another study was conducted to evaluate the efficacy of 5 mW laser irradiation in the treatment of chronic tinnitus, and 66 ears of 45 patients with chronic unilateral or bilateral tinnitus were treated in these studies. Transmeatal low-power (5 mW) laser irradiation was found to be beneficial in the treatment of chronic tinnitus [55]. Many other studies achieved the same results [56].

2.8 Ear canal magnets

According to Takeda, previous studies on the ionization fluctuation of the inner ear on the proteins and phospholipids of hair cell membranes have revealed a potential relationship between ion disorders and tinnitus [57]. Apparently, satisfactory outcomes were achieved with the use of rare-earth magnets in affecting ion disorders and in the treatment of tinnitus. However, it seems that references to these claims do not support them. Takeda's methods include placing a 4 mm diameter circular 1800 G samarium-cobalt magnet between two thin pieces of cotton and against a tympanic membrane 2 mm thick. An uncontrolled, prospective observational study conducted with 50 patients reported an improvement in the ears of 66% of tinnitus patients [57]. This study was not able to demonstrate any beneficial effect on tinnitus with the use of ear canal magnets. No improvement was seen in either minimum loudness match, minimal masking level changes, or subjective changes in tinnitus severity [3, 57]. In a double-blind study by Takeda on tinnitus treatment in 50 patients that involved the placement of rare-earth magnets, no evidence of significant benefits could be provided with this form of treatment [58].

2.9 Ultrasound

Using ultrasound for treating tinnitus was found inadvertently. A patient who underwent ultrasonic examination of the maxillary antrum claimed to have had their tinnitus relieved during the process. Improvement is short term but repeatable. It is known that some types of ultrasound might alter cell morphology, biochemistry, or behavior through hydrodynamic shearing forces produced by characterization activity, or typically, by a significant increase in the temperature [59]. However, the exact mechanism which provides benefits for tinnitus is not known. In a study by Rendell et al., there was no significant difference in the loudness match of tinnitus, grading scales analysis, and the verbal reports of the placebo group and the group treated with ultrasound.

Another study by Carrick et al. demonstrated a distinctly more frequent sense of improvement in patients who have used active devices [3]. This study aimed to determine whether or not a low-dose ultrasound applied to mastoid bone provided subjective improvements in the tinnitus levels of long-term patients.

In another study, 40 patients volunteered to enroll in a double-blind study. They received 10-minute treatment with an ultrasound generator, and then the same placebo device, in two separate visits. Devices were separated randomly during the first visit. In every visit, the patients stated whether tinnitus was completely healed, slightly healed, did not change, or was made worse by the treatment. Forty percent of the patients who completed the study were healed through ultrasound, and 7% through placebo. Low-power ultrasound provided a greater improvement when compared to placebo [60].

2.10 Electromagnetic stimulation

The suppressive effect of electromagnetic stimulation on tinnitus was observed in patients with cochlear implants. Other studies have found a suppressive effect on tinnitus by using direct current stimulation of the cochlea. Stimulation via the round window membrane is the most effective method; however, the suppression lasts only throughout the current flow, and only anodal stimulation is effective. Risks of this treatment include tissue damage and surgery. The three studies conducted have not demonstrated significant benefits over electromagnetic stimulation. Another study by Roland revealed that the active device provided a significant improvement in the symptom score and tinnitus match, and a 9% improvement was seen in the placebo group when compared to 45% of patients treated with electromagnetic stimulation [61].

Results of another study conducted to determine whether or not pulsed electromagnetic stimulation on mastoid bone provided an improvement in tinnitus level of patients with long-standing tinnitus were reported. Fifty-eight patients volunteered for a double-blind, placebo-controlled study. Active and placebo devices were separated randomly in these patients' first visit. At the end of the 1-week treatment, each patient stated whether tinnitus was completely removed, healed, did not change, or was made worse by the treatment. Forty-five percent of the patients who completed the trial showed improvement with the active device. Furthermore, 9% of them reported improvement with the placebo. It is therefore thought that electromagnetic stimulation could be an effective treatment with some tinnitus patients [62].

2.11 Herbal practice

2.11.1 Ginkgo biloba

Ginkgo is a tree that grows in China. The first publication on the use of *Ginkgo biloba* leaves for medical purposes dates back to a 1505 AD text by Liu Wen-Tai called Ben Cao Pin Hue Jing Yaor. The text states that high-quality, standardized extracts derived from the leaves of this tree improved cerebrovascular blood flow and were used to treat cerebral insufficiency, memory disorders, and tinnitus [3].

Ginkgo biloba extract helps minimize the damage induced by free radical accumulation in the cochlea, which is caused by a potent glutamate antagonist acting as a potent antagonist. EGB761 is the most common isolate of *Ginkgo biloba* that increases circulation in the body. It is beneficial for vascular insufficiency and cognitive function [63]. It has been recommended as a mechanism for the treatment of tinnitus by improving blood circulation to the Corti's organ [64]. In a rodent model, even minimal doses of EGB761 provided a statistically significant decrease in behavioral manifestation of tinnitus induced by sodium salicylate toxicity [65].

Reports such as these assert that *Ginkgo biloba*, one of the most ancient herbs, enables significant improvements in patients with tinnitus. Other contradictory studies have not defined any effect for tinnitus [66].

2.11.2 Zinc

Zinc is an important trace element present in all organs, tissues, fluids, and secretions of the body. It is distributed throughout the central nervous system, including the auditory pathway in synapses from the cochlea to the eighth cranial nerve [67]. Zinc is the fundamental component of Cu/Zn superoxide dismutase (SOD). It is important for the proper functioning of more than 300 enzymes, as well as the synthesis and stabilization of deoxyribonucleic acid (DNA), ribonucleic acid (RNA), and proteins. It also plays a structural role in the function of ribosomes and membranes. Otolaryngology-related studies were used to examine the effects of abnormal zinc levels as a cause of anosmia [68] and burning mouth syndrome [69]. Three potential mechanisms relating to tinnitus are linked to zinc [70]: Cochlear Cu/Zn SOD activity, synaptic transmission, and depression. The literature suggests that the prevalence rates of zinc deficiency are more suitable for elderly individuals and individuals with a tinnitus range from 2–69% [70, 71]. Even though not all studies have shown clinically significant results [72, 73], a limited number of studies point to the beneficial effects of zinc on tinnitus [67, 71, 74]. It is possible to improve the overall effect of treatment by classifying tinnitus patients through the measurement of their serum zinc levels.

2.11.3 Melatonin

Melatonin is a hormone produced at night by the pineal gland. Its main function appears to be regulating the sleep–wake cycle. However, not all effects of melatonin have been completely defined [75]. It is readily available as a nonprescription remedy and is widely used to help patients with sleep disorders. Many studies have examined whether or not its use can be connected with tinnitus. In a randomized, prospective, double-blind, placebo-controlled study conducted with 23 patients, melatonin was subjectively reported to be beneficial in tinnitus treatment. Greater benefits were observed with patients with sleep disorders. Other studies have revealed similar results [76–79].

2.11.4 Vitamin B12

There are some reports that show a relationship between vitamin B12 deficiency and auditory pathway disorders. In a study, it was observed that vitamin B12 replacement treatment provided an improvement in the tinnitus of some patients. It was also concluded that vitamin B12 serum levels should be monitored routinely while evaluating chronic tinnitus patients. A potential mechanism in a few cases of severe vitamin B12 deficiency is increased cardiac output, arterial pressure, and anemia caused by vitamin B12 deficiency. This increased flow is perceived as a ringing in the ear. Vitamin B12 deficiency is a potentially treatable cause of pulsatile tinnitus. As another potential mechanism, vitamin B12 is required for the mutase activation of methylmalonyl coenzyme A, which is necessary for myelin synthesis [63]. In this way, cobalamin deficiency may lead to combined peripheral and central nervous system dysfunction.

2.11.5 Garlic

Connections have been made between garlic and some lipid-lowering effects. A few studies have revealed some potential effects of garlic in increasing fibrinolytic activity and lowering blood pressure [80]. It is believed that the main effects of garlic on tinnitus are due to its potential of improving blood flow to the cochlear artery by reducing plaque formation, stabilizing blood pressure, and increasing the antioxidant capacity of the blood. This effect is only theoretical, and there are therefore no scientific studies which examine the potential effects of garlic on tinnitus.

2.12 Herbal mixtures

The diversity and lack of standardization in terms of the preparation of herbal treatments' diversity make it almost impossible to come to a meaningful conclusion regarding their efficacy. No study has yet been conducted using scientific methodology, and so any claims about the benefits of herbal treatments are merely anecdotal.

2.12.1 Traditional Korean medicine and traditional Chinese medicine

The use of the herbal medicines bojungikgitang and banhabaekchulchonmatang in the treatment of tinnitus has its origins in the principles of traditional Korean medicine. Generally, tinnitus is thought to develop due to dysfunctional irregularities in the intestines and visceral organs. Bojungikgitang is used in the treatment of chi energy deficiency, and banhabaekchulchonmatang is used to treat gallbladder problems, which are thought to be associated with tinnitus. These two remedies are very common in Korea and have been approved by the Korea Food and Drug Administration as herbal medications in adults for the treatment of tinnitus.

Despite the lack of scientifically solid studies, there are anecdotal reports that suggest that traditional Chinese medicine is successful in relieving tinnitus. Er Ming Fang (EMF01) is a Chinese herbal mixture that contains various different herbs. Research studies have not demonstrated any benefits with salicylate-induced tinnitus in rats [81].

Yokukansan is an herbal medicine used in traditional Japanese medicine. It is thought to be an effective treatment for undifferentiated somatoform tinnitus [82].

2.13 Aromatherapy

Tinnitus patients are sometimes attracted to nontraditional or alternative treatments. However, there is no convincing evidence of the efficacy of any complementary therapy in the treatment of tinnitus [83]. However, considering the lack of traditional treatment options, and the placebo reaction which is observed with tinnitus, low-risk therapies such as aromatherapy should not be dismissed, and they are often sought by patients.

NCCAM classifications	CAM therapies	
Alternative medical systems	Acupuncture	Acupuncture by experienced and licensed practitioners might be an option for tinnitus patients, which can help decrease the intensity of tinnitus and improve the quality of life for patients. This treatment tends to only be for the short term. Nonetheless, it remains a possible treatment for patients and is a relatively safe procedure for patients to consider
	Homeopathy	In homeopathy, through the use of a "satisfying dose" for treatment purposes, homeopathic principles may use large "homeopathic" doses of a substance that triggers a symptom in order to stimulate a physiological reaction against the symptoms, thereby eliminating the discomfort. This remedy may be beneficial to a person who has tinnitus with associated deafness
	Hyperbaric oxygen treatment	Hyperbaric oxygen (HBO) treatment as an alternative therapy when standard treatments fail. HBO treatment should be initiated at the earliest opportunity, particularly in tinnitus cases that are accompanied by a sudden loss in hearing. Treatment success in case of sudden deafness depends on the rapid application of HBO
Mind–body medicine	Yoga, hypnosis, biofeedback, neurofeedback, imagery	Mind–body medicines have been associated with low levels of stress and anxiety and a high quality of life. These therapies can be very effective in coping with the psychological aspects of tinnitus such as anger, stress, and anxiety. The main benefit of mind–body treatments is the fact that they can provide relief and sense of relaxation, making tinnitus more bearable
Biologically-based therapies	Dietary and herbal supplements Aromatherapy Chinese herbal medicine Chinese medicine Dietary medicine Clinical nutrition including multivitamins and minerals Western herbal medicine	The use of biologically based therapies to treat tinnitus is common, particularly with *Ginkgo biloba*, magnesium, melatonin, vitamin B12, and zinc. It is likely that some supplements will help with sleep for some patients. However, they are generally not effective, and many produced adverse effects. Dietary supplements could have a positive outcome on tinnitus reactions in some people. These therapies for chronic tinnitus may exert additional efficacy by improving psychological sensation of tinnitus and sleep quality. Future randomized controlled double-blind studies should be performed to elucidate its efficacy
Manipulative and body-based methods	Magnet/laser therapy	Application of magnets and ultrasound has been found to be placebo therapies for tinnitus or to have limited scientific supports for their effectiveness. Additional studies are needed
Energy therapies	Bioalan (Bioelectromagnetics)	Recent and ongoing research studies have attempted to assess whether transcranial magnetic stimulation could be an effective tinnitus treatment. This application is based on the thought that tinnitus is associated with an irregular activation of the temporoparietal cortex (a part of the brain) and thus that disturbing this irregular activation could result in transient reduction of tinnitus

Table 1.
The National Center for Complementary and Alternative Medicine (NCCAM) complementary and alternative treatments [87].

The basis of holistic and complementary treatments is primarily the fact that they reduce the symptoms of patients or minimize the discomfort associated with such symptoms. Aromatherapy, which is the most common alternative approach, requires a combination of essential oils and massage to reduce the symptoms of the disorder and make the patient feel better.

Aromatherapy uses frankincense, which dates back to ancient Babylon, and various oil groups (e.g., rowan, chamomile, frankincense, lavender, and mint) [84]. Hippocrates suggested that the way to health was to have aromatic baths and massages. It is known that virgin cedarwood oil was used for hygienic purposes 5000 years ago by the Egyptians [85]. Both the lavender plant and its essential oil were used by abbess Hildegard of Bingen at the beginning of the twelfth century. It is thought that the essential oils of turpentine, cinnamon, frankincense, juniper, rose, and sage were known and used in the fifteenth century [84].

According to the results of this study, it is considered that the majority of patients benefited from aromatherapy, while the benefits were shown to be non-specific rather than directly associated with tinnitus. Patients reported that the aromatherapy helped them to relax and that other somatic symptoms were eased.

Even though aromatherapy has a negative effect on being able to ignore tinnitus, relaxation was also seen to be advantageous in other studies on relaxation approaches [86].

A list of The National Center for Complementary and Alternative Medicine (NCCAM) complementary and alternative treatments can be found in **Table 1**.

3. Conclusion

Tinnitus does not have an established treatment as its pathophysiology has not been completely understood. Patients who cannot sufficiently benefit from medical treatments often try complementary and alternative treatments. In the studies conducted, it was demonstrated that such approaches provided benefits for some tinnitus patients. Through a holistic approach combined with medical know-how, patients can gain control over their problems, decrease, or even eliminate the effects of these problems. For that reason, the prevalence and acceptance of nontraditional approaches for tinnitus have increased among both patients and practitioners. Consequently, it is recommended that patients who cannot sufficiently benefit from medical treatments be referred to acknowledged experts for complementary and alternative treatments.

Author details

Ismail Aytaç
Medical Faculty, Department of Otolaryngology, Gaziantep University, Gaziantep, Turkey

*Address all correspondence to: dr.iaytac@gmail.com

IntechOpen

References

[1] Pinto PCL, Sanchez TG, Tomita S. Avaliação da relação entre severidade do zumbido e perda auditiva, sexo e idade do paciente. Brazilian Journal of Otorhinolaryngology. 2010;**76**:18-24

[2] Norena AJ. An integrative model of tinnitus based on a central gain controlling neural sensitivity. Neuroscience and Biobehavioral Reviews. 2011;**35**:1089-1109

[3] Meehan T, Eisenhut M, Stephens D. A review of alternative treatments for tinnitus. Audiological Medicine. 2004;**2**(1):74-82

[4] Okada DM, Onishi ET, Chami FI, Borin A, Cassola N, Guerreiro VM. Acupuncture for tinnitus immediate relief. Brazilian Journal of Otorhinolaryngology. 2006;**72**:182-186

[5] Kim JI, Choi JY, Lee DH, Choi TY, Lee MS, Ernst E. Acupuncture for the treatment of tinnitus: A systematic review of randomized clinical trials. BMC Complementary and Alternative Medicine. 2012;**12**:97

[6] Tano SS, Schultz AR, Borges R, Marchiori LLDM. Effectiveness of acupuncture therapy as treatment for tinnitus: A randomized controlled trial. Brazilian Journal of Otorhinolaryngology. 2016;**82**(4):458-465

[7] Mason S, Tovey P, Long AF. Evaluating complementary medicine: Methodological challenges of randomised controlled trials. British Medical Journal. 2002;**325**:832-834

[8] Dobie R. A review of randomised clinical trials in tinnitus. The Laryngoscope. 1999;**109**:1202-1211

[9] Silencing Tinnitus. BPJ:47. [Internet]. 2012. Available from: https://bpac.org. nz/BPJ/2012/october/docs/bpj_47_ tinnitus_pages_28-37.pdf [Accessed: 2018-07-04]

[10] Chami FAI. A utilização da acupuntura em pacientes portadores de zumbido. In: Lovise, editor. Zumbido: Avaliação, Diagnóstico e Reabilitação-Abordagens atuais; 2004. p. 113

[11] Ernst E, White AR. Prospective studies of the safety of acupuncture: A systematic review. The American Journal of Medicine. 2001;**110**(6):481-485

[12] Maciocia G. Os fundamentos da medicina chinesa: um textoabrangente para acupunturistas e fitoterapeutas. 2nd ed. Roca: SãoPaulo; 2007

[13] Yamamura Y. Acupuntura tradicional: A arte de inserir. 2nd ed. São Paulo: Roca; 2004

[14] Azevedo RFD, Chiari BM, Okada DM, Onishi ET. Efeito da acupuntura sobre as emissões otoacústicas de pacientes com zumbido. Brazilian Journal of Otorhinolaryngology. 2007;**73**:599-607

[15] Hao JJ, Cheng W, Liu M, Li H, Lu X, Sun Z. Treatment of multiple sclerosis with Chinese scalp acupuncture. Global Advances in Health and Medicine. 2013;**2**:8-13

[16] Kiyoshita Y. Acupuncture treatment of tinnitus: Evaluation of its efficacy by objective methods. Otolaryngology and Head and Neck Surgery. 1990;**62**:351-357

[17] Vilholm OJ, Moller K, Jorgensen K. Effect of traditional Chinese acupuncture on severe tinnitus: A double-blind, placebo-controlled, clinical investigation with open therapeutic control. British Journal of Audiology. 1998;**32**(3):197-204

[18] Martinez-Devesa P, Waddel A, Perera R, Theodoulou M. Cognitive behavioral therapy for tinnitus. Cochrane Database Systematic Reviews. PLoS One. 2007;**1**:1-22

[19] Kim SD. Effects of yogic exercises on life stress and blood glucose levels in nursing students. Journal of Physical Therapy Science. 2014;**26**(12):2003-2006

[20] Vorkapic CF, Rangé B. Reducing the symptomatology of panic disorder: The effects of a yoga program alone and in combination with cognitive-behavioral therapy. Frontiers in Psychiatry. 2014;**5**(5):177

[21] Farifteh S, Mohammadi-Aria A, Kiamanesh A, Mofid B. The impact of laughter yoga on the stress of cancer patients before chemotherapy. Iranian Journal of Cancer Prevention. 2014;**7**(4):179-183

[22] Wang D, Hagins M. Perceived benefits of yoga among urban school students: A qualitative analysis. Evidence-based Complementary and Alternative Medicine. 2016;**2016**:8725654. DOI: 10.1155/2016/8725654

[23] Köksoy S, Eti CM, Karataş M, Vayisoglu Y. The effects of yoga in patients suffering from subjective tinnitus. International Archives of Otorhinolaryngology. 2018;**22**(1):9-13

[24] Gilbert C, Moss D. Biofeedback and biological monitoring. In: Moss D, McGrady A, Davies T, Wickramasekera I, editors. Handbook of Mind-Body Medicine for Primary Care. Thousand Oaks CA: Sage; 2003. pp. 109-122

[25] Sherman RA. Pain Assessment & Intervention: From a Psychophysiological Perspective. Wheat Ridge, CO: Association for Applied Psychophysiology and Biofeedback; 2004

[26] Seaward B. Managing Stress: Principles and Strategies for Health and Wellbeing. Sudbury, MA: Jones and Bartlett Publishers; 2006

[27] Norena A, Micheyl C, Chery-Croze S, Collet L. Psychoacoustic characterization of the tinnitus spectrum: Implications for the underlying mechanisms of tinnitus. Audiology & Neuro-Otology. 2002;**7**:358-369

[28] Weisz N, Hartmann T, Dohrmann K, Schlee W, Norena A. High-frequency tinnitus without hearing loss does not mean absence of deafferentation. Hearing Research. 2006;**222**:108-114

[29] Elbert T, Heim S. A light and a dark side. Nature. 2001;**411**:139

[30] Moller AR. The role of neural plasticity in tinnitus. Progress in Brain Research. 2007;**166**:37-45

[31] Weisz N, Moratti S, Meinzer M, Dohrmann K, Elbert T. Tinnitus perception and distress is related to abnormal spontaneous brain activity as measured by magnetoencephalography. PLoS Medicine. 2005;**2**:e153

[32] Lehtela L, Salmelin R, Hari R. Evidence for reactive magnetic 10 Hz rhythm in the human auditory cortex. Neuroscience Letters. 1997;**222**:111-114

[33] Fuchs T, Birbaumer N, Lutzenberger W, Gruzelier JH, Kaiser J. Neurofeedback treatment for attention-deficit/hyperactivity disorder in children: A comparison with methylphenidate. Applied Psychophysiology and Biofeedback. 2003;**28**:1-12

[34] Landis B, Landis E. Is biofeedback effective for chronic tinnitus? An intensive study with seven subjects. American Journal of Otolaryngology. 1992;**13**:349-356

[35] Weise C, Heinecke K, Rief W. Biofeedback-based behavioral treatment for chronic tinnitus: Results of a randomized controlled trial. Journal of Consulting and Clinical Psychology. 2008;**76**:1046-1057

[36] Weise C, Heinecke K, Rief W. Stability of physiological variables in chronic tinnitus sufferers. Applied Psychophysiology and Biofeedback. 2008;**33**:149-159

[37] Gosepath K, Nafe B, Ziegler E, Mann WJ. Neurofeedback in therapy of tinnitus. HNO. 2001;**49**:29-35

[38] Schenk S, Lamm K, Gundel H, Ladwig KH. Neurofeedback-based EEG alpha and EEG beta training. Effectiveness in patients with chronically decompensated tinnitus. HNO. 2005;**53**:29-37

[39] Schlee W, Hartmann T, Langguth B, Weisz N. Abnormal resting state cortical coupling in chronic tinnitus. BMC Neuroscience. 2009;**10**:11

[40] Crocetti A, Forti S, Del Bo L. Neurofeedback for subjective tinnitus patients. Auris, Nasus, Larynx. 2011;**38**(6):735-738

[41] Dohrmann K, Elbert T, Schlee W, Weisz N. Tuning the tinnitus percept by modification of synchronous brain activity. Restorative Neurology and Neuroscience. 2007;**25**:371-378

[42] Tinnitus. [Internet]. 2018. Available from: https://www.hypnotherapy-directory.org.uk/articles/tinnitus.html [Accessed: 2018-07-04]

[43] Matthews W. Ericksonian approaches to hypnosis and therapy: Where are we now? The International Journal of Clinical and Experimental Hypnosis. 2000;**48**(4):418-426

[44] Gonsalkorale WM, Miller V, Afzal A, Whorwell PJ. Long term benefits of hypnotherapy for irritable bowel syndrome. Gut. 2003;**52**:1623-1629

[45] Saadat H, Drummond-Lewis J, Maranets I, et al. Hypnosis reduces preoperative anxiety in adult patients. Anesthesia and Analgesia. 2006;**102**(5):1394-1396

[46] Kirsch I, Montgomery G, Sapirstein G. Hypnosis as an adjunct to cognitive-behavioral psychotherapy: A metaanalysis. Journal of Consulting and Clinical Psychology. 1995;**63**(2):214-220

[47] Woldorff MG, Gallen CC, Hampson SA, et al. Modulation of early sensory processing in human auditory cortex during auditory selective attention. Proceedings of the National Academy of Sciences of the United States of America. 1993;**90**:8722-8726

[48] Grady CL, Van Meter JW, Maisog JM, Pietrini P, Krasuski J, Rauschecker JP. Attention related modulation of activity in primary and secondary auditory cortex. Neuroreport. 1997;**8**(11):2511-2516

[49] Cope TE. Clinical hypnosis for the alleviation of tinnitus. The International Tinnitus Journal. 2008;**14**(2):135-138

[50] Baldwin TM. Tinnitus, a military epidemic: Is hyperbaric oxygen therapy the answer? Journal of Special Operations Medicine: A Peer Reviewed Journal for SOF Medical Professionals. 2009;**9**(3):33-43

[51] Bohmer D. Treating tinnitus with hyperbaric oxygenation. The International Tinnitus Journal. 1997;**3**(2)

[52] Simpson JJ, Donaldson I, Davies WE. Use of homeopathy in the treatment of tinnitus. British Journal of Audiology. 1998;**32**(4):227-233

[53] Shiomi Y, Takahashi H, Honjo I, Kojima H, Naito Y, Fujiki N. Efficacy of

transmeatal low power laser irradiation on tinnitus: A preliminary report. Auris, Nasus, Larynx. 1997;**24**(1):39-42

[54] Nakashima T, Ueda H, Misawa H, Suzuki T, Tominaga M, Ito A, et al. Transmeatal low-power laser irradiation for tinnitus. Otology & Neurotology. 2002;**23**(3):296-300

[55] Gungor A, Dogru S, Cincik H, Erkul E, Poyrazoglu E. Effectiveness of transmeatal low power laser irradiation for chronic tinnitus. The Journal of Laryngology & Otology. 2008;**122**(5):447-451

[56] Teggi R, Bellini C, Piccioni LO, Palonta F, Bussi M. Transmeatal low-level laser therapy for chronic tinnitus with cochlear dysfunction. Audiology and Neurotology. 2009;**14**(2):115-120

[57] Takeda H. Magnetic therapy for tinnitus. Otologia Fukuoka. 1987;**33**:700-706

[58] Coles R, Bradley P, Donaldson I, Dingle A. A trial of tinnitus therapy with ear-canal magnets. Clinical Otolaryngology and Allied Sciences. 1991;**16**(4):371-372

[59] Rendell R, Carrick D, Fielder C, Callaghan D, Thomas K. Low-powered ultrasound in the inhibition of tinnitus. British Journal of Audiology. 1987;**21**:289-293

[60] Carrick DG, Davies WM, Fielder CP, Bihari J. Low-powered ultrasound in the treatment of tinnitus: A pilot study. British Journal of Audiology. 1986;**20**(2):153-155

[61] Fiedler SC, Pilkington H, Willatt DJ. Electromagnetic stimulation as a treatment of tinnitus: A further study. Clinical Otolaryngology. 1998;**23**:270

[62] Roland NJ, Hughes JB, Daley MB, Cook JA, Jones AS, McCormick MS. Electromagnetic stimulation as a

treatment of tinnitus: A pilot study. Clinical Otolaryngology and Allied Sciences. 1993;**18**(4):278-281

[63] Seidman MD, Babu S. Alternative medications and other treatments for tinnitus: Facts from fiction. Otolaryngologic Clinics of North America. 2003;**36**(2):359-381

[64] Patterson MB, Balough BJ. Review of pharmacological therapy for tinnitus. The International Tinnitus Journal. 2006;**12**(2):149-160

[65] Jastreboff PJ, Zhou S, Jastreboff MM, Kwapisz U, Gryczynska U. Attenuation of salicylate-induced tinnitus by Ginkgo biloba extract in rats. Audiology and Neurotology. 1997;**2**(4):197-212

[66] Drew S, Davies E. Effectiveness of Ginkgo biloba in treating tinnitus: Double blind, placebo controlled trial. British Medical Journal. 2001;**322**(7278):73-78

[67] Shambaugh GE Jr. Zinc for tinnitus, imbalance, and hearing loss in the elderly. The American Journal of Otology. 1986;**7**(6):476-477

[68] Alexander TH, Davidson TM. Intranasal zinc and anosmia: The zinc-induced anosmia syndrome. The Laryngoscope. 2006;**116**(2): 217-220

[69] Cho GS, Han MW, Lee B, et al. Zinc deficiency may be a cause of burning mouth syndrome as zinc replacement therapy has therapeutic effects. Journal of Oral Pathology & Medicine. 2010;**39**(9):722-727

[70] Coelho CB, Tyler R, Hansen M. Zinc as a possible treatment for tinnitus. Progress in Brain Research. 2007;**166**:279-285

[71] Arda HN, Tuncel U, Akdogan O, Ozluoglu LN. The role of zinc in the

treatment of tinnitus. Otology & Neurotology. 2003;**24**(1):86-89

[72] Paaske PB, Kiems G, Pedersen CB, Sam ILK. Zinc in the management of tinnitus. Placebo-controlled trial. The Annals of Otology, Rhinology, and Laryngology. 1991;**100**(8):647-649

[73] Yetiser S, Tosun F, Satar B, Arslanhan M, Akcam T, Ozkaptan Y. The role of zinc in management of tinnitus. Auris, Nasus, Larynx. 2002;**29**(4):329-333

[74] Ochi K, Ohashi T, Kinoshita H, et al. The serum zinc level in patients with tinnitus and the effect of zinc treatment. Nihon Jibiinkoka Gakkai Kaiho. 1997;**100**(9):915-919

[75] Pirodda A, Raimondi MC, Ferri GG. Exploring the reasons why melatonin can improve tinnitus. Medical Hypotheses. 2010;**75**(2):190-191

[76] Hurtuk A, Dome C, Holloman CH, Wolfe K, Welling DB, Dodson EE, et al. Melatonin: Can it stop the ringing? The Annals of Otology, Rhinology, and Laryngology. 2011;**120**(7):433-440

[77] Lopez-Gonzalez MA, Santiago AM, Esteban-Ortega F. Sulpiride and melatonin decrease tinnitus perception modulating the auditolimbic dopaminergic pathway. The Journal of Otolaryngology. 2007;**36**(4):213-219

[78] Megwalu UC, Finnell JE, Piccirillo JF. The effects of melatonin on tinnitus and sleep. Otolaryngology and Head and Neck Surgery. 2006;**134**(2):210-213

[79] Seabra ML, Bignotto M, Pinto LR Jr, Tufik S. Randomized, double-blind clinical trial, controlled with placebo, of the toxicology of chronic melatonin treatment. Journal of Pineal Research. 2000;**29**(4):193-200

[80] FLinde K, ter Riet G, Hondras M, et al. Systematic reviews of complementary therapies—An annotated bibliography. Part 2: Herbal medicine. BMC Complementary and Alternative Medicine. 2001;**1**:5

[81] Zheng Y, Vagal S, Zhu XX, et al. The effects of the Chinese herbal medicine EMF01 on salicylate induced tinnitus in rats. Journal of Ethnopharmacology. 2010;**128**(2):545-548

[82] Okamoto H, Okami T, Ikeda M, Takeuchi T. Effects of Yokukansan on undifferentiated somatoform disorder with tinnitus. European Psychiatry. 2005;**20**(1):74-75

[83] Moss C. The desktop guide to complementary and alternative medicine: An evidence-based approach. Journal of the Royal Society of Medicine. 2001:650-651 p

[84] Meehan T, Stephens D, Wilson C, Lewis C. Aromatherapy in tinnitus: A pilot study. Audiological Medicine. 2003;**1**(2):144-147

[85] Robertshawe P, Price S, Price L. Aromatherapy for health professionals. Journal of the Australian Traditional-Medicine Society. 2009;**15**(2):101-102

[86] Davies S, McKenna L, Hallam RS. Relaxation and cognitive therapy: A controlled trial in chronic tinnitus. Psychology and Health. 1995;**10**(2):129-143

[87] Integrative Health. [Internet]. Available from: https://nccih.nih.gov/health/integrative-health [Accessed: 2018-11-04-15]

www.ingramcontent.com/pod-product-compliance
Lightning Source LLC
Chambersburg PA
CBHW081241190326
41458CB00016B/5873